Radiology plays a central role in diagnosis, management and ‹
of a patient's condition. The increasing importance of radiolog
medicine has led to the inclusion of the subject in medical school curricula
worldwide. Most radiology teaching for medical students is conducted
around films of real patients on the ward or in tutorial groups within the
radiology department itself and, by reflecting this method of learning, the
approach of this book will be familiar to students studying radiology at
undergraduate level. The book adopts a systemic approach to cover the
commonest clinical problems that are encountered on the wards, in tutorials
and in examinations. Clear radiographs are each presented with brief reports
and an accompanying discussion of the diagnosis, differential diagnosis and
potential further investigations. This new edition is enhanced with many
new images, and all are now clearly labelled and arrowed to highlight
significant diagnostic features.

Reviews of first edition

'Radiology conjures up a plethora of reactions in medical students, from an
inquisitive interest to pure hatred. Most share one thing in common, a wish
to be somewhere else when a clinician asks you to present and interpret a
radiological image. Those moments of motionless dread need not be so;
Radiology made easy is here to help us all! This book is a splendid overview
of a host of common imaging techniques and findings, including plain
radiography, magnetic resonance imaging, computed tomography, and
ultrasound.'
Student BMJ

This book is dedicated to

My mother and father
My wife Tina
My daughters, Shonali and Shiuli
My students past, present and future

Radiology

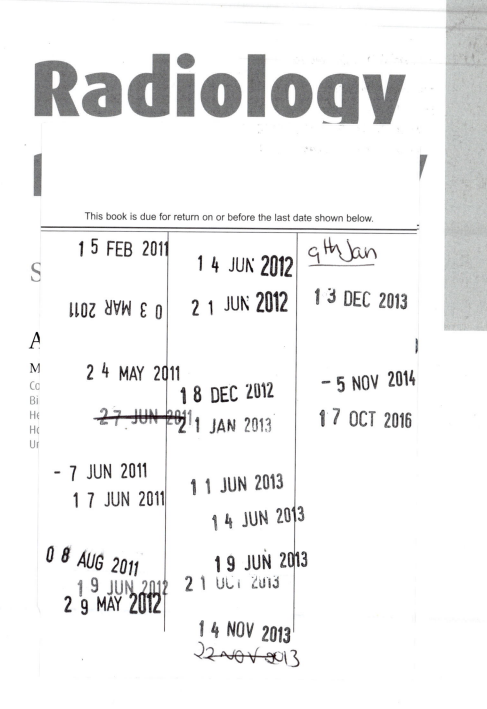

This book is due for return on or before the last date shown below.

1 5 FEB 2011

1 4 JUN 2012   9th Jan

0 3 MAR 2011   2 1 JUN 2012   1 3 DEC 2013

2 4 MAY 2011
                     1 8 DEC 2012   - 5 NOV 2014
27 JUN 2011   2 1 JAN 2013   1 7 OCT 2016

- 7 JUN 2011
  1 7 JUN 2011   1 1 JUN 2013

                      1 4 JUN 2013

0 8 AUG 2011   1 9 JUN 2013
  1 9 JUN 2012   2 1 OCT 2013
  2 9 MAY 2012

                      1 4 NOV 2013
                      22 NOV 2013

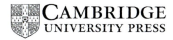
CAMBRIDGE
UNIVERSITY PRESS

CAMBRIDGE UNIVERSITY PRESS

Cambridge, New York, Melbourne, Madrid, Cape Town, Singapore, São Paulo

CAMBRIDGE UNIVERSITY PRESS

The Edinburgh Building, Cambridge CB2 2RU, UK

Published in the United States of America by Cambridge University Press, New York

www.cambridge.org
Information on this title: www.cambridge.org/9780521672306

First published 1999
Second edition published 2006

Printed in the United Kingdom at the University Press, Cambridge

A catalogue record for this publication is available from the British Library

Library of Congress Cataloguing in Publication data

ISBN   PB   0-521-67635-5

Every effort has been made in preparing this publication to provide accurate and up-to-date
information which is in accord with accepted standards and practice at the time of publication.
Although case histories are drawn from actual cases, every effort has been made to disguise the
identities of the individuals involved. Nevertheless, the authors, editors and publishers can make
no warranties that the information contained herein is totally free from error, not least because
clinical standards are constantly changing through research and regulation. The authors, editors
and publishers therefore disclaim all liability for direct or consequential damages resulting from
the use of material contained in this publication. Readers are strongly advised to pay careful
attention to information provided by the manufacturer of any drugs or equipment that they
plan to use.

Contents

Introduction

Section A ■ The chest

Section B ■ Gastrointestinal system

Section C ■ The central nervous system

Section D ■ Bone

Section E ■ Renal, gynaecological and vascular systems

Preface

In the last 20 years radiology has undergone rapid advancement and today it often plays a central role in diagnosis, management and even treatment of a patient's problems. The increasing importance of radiology in clinical medicine has led to the inclusion of the subject in medical school curricula worldwide. Most radiology teaching for medical students is conducted around films of patients on the ward or in more structured groups in a tutorial format, usually in the radiology department.

In this book I have covered some of the commonest clinical problems encountered on the wards, in tutorials and in examinations. The radiographs are presented with brief reports and discussion on different diagnoses and further investigations. The book is written in a style more familiar to a radiology tutorial than a didactic comprehensive text. As such it should prove a useful accompaniment for radiology tutorials at medical schools and will also serve as an introduction to the subject. The book may also be useful to junior doctors and as a revision aide for higher general medical exams.

Arpan K. Banerjee
June, 1999
Birmingham

Preface to second edition

Over the last 5 years, since the publication of the first edition of this well received text book, radiology has moved swiftly into the 21st century. The main technological advances include the more widespread use of multislice CT scanners which enable faster and more rapid CT scanning. In addition clinical PET is now coming of age. Departments in the western world are now going digital. The basics of radiology however remain essentially unchanged. Radiology will always primarily be concerned with providing a diagnosis on patients and then hopefully modern radiological techniques will enable more minimally invasive methods of treatment. Radiology remains as important to good clinical care as it always has been.

In the second edition of this book I have updated some of the key concepts of radiology and have also upgraded several of the images and introduced arrows on the radiographs to facilitate learning. A number of new images are also included. I hope that the book will continue to be a useful accompaniment for radiology tutorials at medical schools and will also serve as a useful introductory text book for both undergraduate and post graduate medical students and allied healthcare professionals.

April 2005

Acknowledgements

Thanks are due to the following for their help with this project:

The Medical Illustration Department at the Birmingham Heartlands Hospital
My clinical colleagues for sending the patients for the investigations
My radiology colleagues who conducted some of the procedures illustrated
The radiographers of Heartlands and Solihull Hospitals without whom the patients could not have been investigated

Geoff Nuttall of Greenwich Medical Media for the opportunity to start the project, Gavin Smith for his continued support and Nora Naughton for her help with the production

Finally, my wife for her patience while the book was being written and my daughters Shonali and Shiuli for providing me with inspiration for the future.

April 2005

List of abbreviated figure captions

Section A: The chest

Section B: Gastrointestinal system

Introduction to the chest X-ray

How the radiograph is taken

The standard view is the postero-anterior (PA) view with the patient in full inspiration. The patient stands erect with the anterior chest wall against the film cassette and the X-ray beam enters from behind. If the patient cannot stand, an antero-posterior (AP) film is taken but this magnifies the cardiac and mediastinal shadows.

How to analyse the chest film

- Check the name
- Check the patient's gender
- Check left and right markers
- Check for extra objects on the radiograph
  - central line
  - endotracheal tube
  - electrocardiogram (ECG) leads
  - chest drains
  - pacemaker, etc.
- Check centring of film. Medial ends of the clavicle should be equidistant from the spinous process of the vertebrae
- Assess penetration of the film. The lower thoracic vertebrae should be visible through the heart shadow with ideal penetration
- Check lung volumes. Midpoint of right hemi-diaphragm should be between the anterior ends of the fifth and seventh ribs
- Look at the lungs
  - check the pulmonary vascular pattern and tissues
  - check hila (the hilar point is the junction of the upper lobe veins and basal pulmonary arteries)
  - check the costophrenic regions
  - the lung is divided into upper, mid- and lower zones demarcated by the anterior ends of the second and fourth ribs
- Review the blind spots
  - apices
  - retrosternal region
  - retrocardiac region
- Look at the mediastinum
  - check that the trachea is central and patent
  - check the left and right heart border

- assess heart size. The ratio of the heart diameter to thoracic diameter (cardiothoracic ratio) should be <0.55
- Look at the soft tissues and bones – check under diaphragm for free intra-peritoneal air

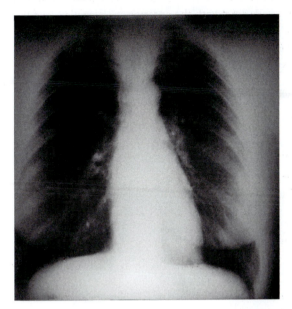

Fig. A1. Normal chest radiograph in a female patient.

This patient has had a long history of hypertension.

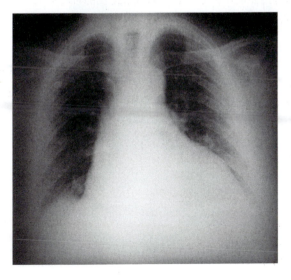

Fig. A2. PA chest radiograph showing an enlarged cardiac diameter. There is no evidence of any upper lobe blood diversion or any pleural effusion. The hila appear normal. No lung parenchymal abnormality is demonstrated on this film.

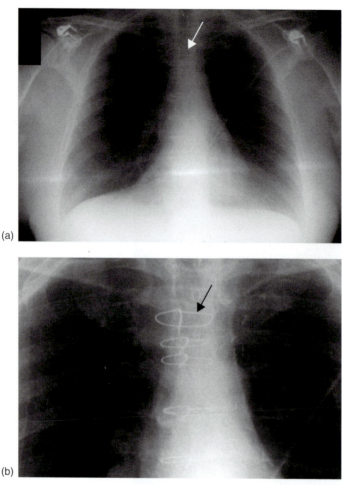

(a)

(b)

Fig. A3. (a) Chest radiograph showing median sternotomy sutures (see arrow) in addition to cardiomegaly. (b) Close-up of sternal region on chest radiograph showing sternotomy sutures and coronary bypass graft clips (see arrow).

Conclusion

- The appearances are those of cardiomegaly.
- The patient has had a recent cardiac operation.

Further in

- Echo (ultra
  ular functi
- Nuclear m
- Angiograph

Causes of I

- Heart failu
- Mitral sten
- Lymphangi
- Pneumocor

 Pul

Pulmonary oed

Causes

- Heart failure,
- Fluid overloa
- Hypoprotein
- Drug reaction
- Poisons, e.g. s
- Cerebrovascu
- Radiotherapy
- Adult respirat
- Drowning

Cardiomegaly

In a PA chest film it is always important to assess heart size, usually assessed as the cardiothoracic ratio, which is the ratio of the maximum cardiac diameter divided by the maximum internal diameter of the chest. This ratio ranges from 0.45 to 0.55 in the normal population. A ratio >0.55 is suggestive of cardiomegaly. Cardiac size can be assessed on serial films to look for a change in size over a time.

Enlargement of individual chambers produce the following signs:

- Left atrium
  - double right heart contour
  - splaying of bronchi
  - posterior bulge on lateral chest radiograph
- Right atrium – prominent right heart border
- Right ventricle
  - upward displacement of cardiac apex
  - anterior bulge on lateral chest radiograph
- Left ventricle – prominent left heart border

Causes of cardiomegaly

- Left ventricular failure
- Mixed mitral valve disease
- Hypertension
- Cardiomyopathy
- Pericardial effusion

Further imaging investigations

- Echocardiography
- Computed tomographic (CT) scanning
- Angiography/ventriculography to assess coronary artery anatomy and cardiac function

Causes

- Trauma (penetrating injury to the lungs)
- Spontaneous, especially in young men
- Emphysema (rupture of bulla)
- AIDS

Signs on chest radiograph

- A line of pleura forming the lung edge clearly separated from the chest wall by air
- No lung markings, e.g. vessels, in this region
- Sign seen best on expiratory film, especially if pneumothorax is small
- In the presence of a pleural effusion a pneumothorax (occurring, for instance, after a pleural aspiration) will cause an air/fluid level (hydropneumothorax)

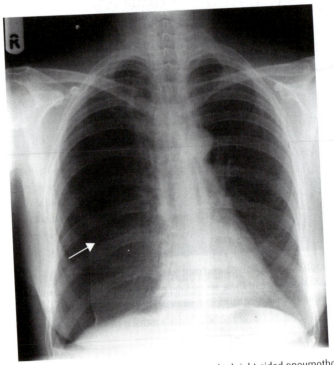

Fig. A15. Chest radiograph showing a less marked right-sided pneumothorax with the pleural line visible on the right separated by air from the chest wall (arrow). A pneumothorax is caused by air entering the pleural cavity.

Fig. A7. Th
In additio
pulmonar

Signs

- Cardic
- Uppe
- Kerley
  ery in
- Pleura
- Interst
- 'Bat's

This patient was a smoker and presented with haemoptysis.

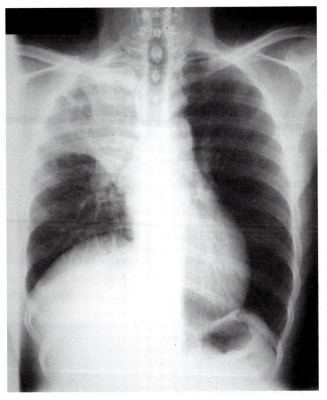

Fig. A16. Chest radiograph showing loss of volume in the right lung. In addition, there is opacification in the right upper zones with elevation of the horizontal fissure. Also, there appears to be a right hilar mass. There is no significant mediastinal shift. The left lung appears normal. Heart size is also normal. The features noted in the right lung are those of right upper lobe collapse, which is almost certainly secondary in this case to a tumour involving the origin of the right upper lobe at the level of the hilum.

Pulmonary collapse

Pulmonary collapse or atelectasis is the loss of volume in a lobe of the lung (or whole lung) caused by obstruction to flow of air. Air in the alveoli is absorbed and because no further air enters the alveoli due to obstruction, the lung tissue collapses and becomes more opaque.

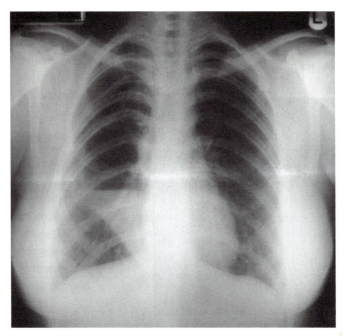

Fig. A19. Radiograph showing a 'wedge-shaped' shadowing adjacent to the right heart border with a clear hemi-diaphragm seen. This is due to a right middle lobe collapse.

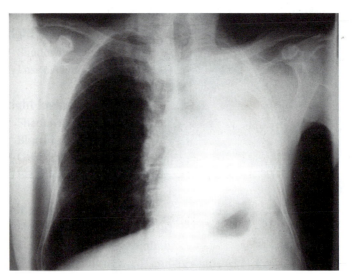

Fig. A20. Radiograph showing a complete opacification of the left lung due to complete obstruction of the left main bronchus and distal collapse of the left lung.

This patient presented for a routine chest radiograph.

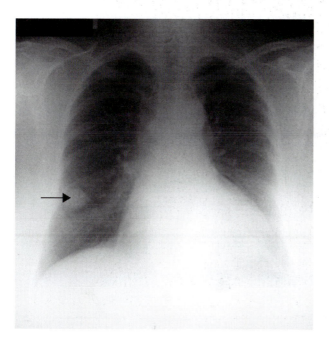

Fig. A21. Heart size is within normal limits. In the right lung there is a 2 cm well-defined mass seen in the right lower zone (arrow). The mass is not abutting the periphery of the thorax; it is not eroding a rib; it is smooth and not spiculated and has no evidence of any calcification within it. There is no evidence of any hilar involvement. No other nodules are seen in the rest of the lungs. The bones appear normal. Appearances are suspicious of a carcinoma of the bronchus.

Pulmonary nodule

The diagnosis and investigation of a solitary pulmonary nodule with no other associated abnormalities is a common clinical problem (Fig. A21).

Common causes of a solitary pulmonary nodule

- Carcinoma of bronchus
- Benign lung tumour, e.g. hamartoma
- Granuloma, e.g. tuberculoma
- Metastasis

Do the following when faced with a solitary pulmonary nodule

- Look and compare with old films to see if the lesion has changed
- Look for calcification (calcified lesions are more likely to be benign). Calcification, however, does not exclude tumour
- Measure its size. If >3 cm it is more likely to be a tumour
- Look at its shape. If ill-defined or spiculated consider a malignancy
- Look for invasion of the ribs
- Look for cavitation
- Look carefully at hila for nodes

Further tests

- Bronchoscopy and biopsy
- CT scan of chest/CT guided biopsy

Causes of multiple pulmonary nodules

- Metastases
- Abscesses
- Wegener's granulomatosis
- Rheumatoid nodules
- Pneumoconiosis

This patient presented with cough, weight loss and tingling in his hands. He was also clubbed.

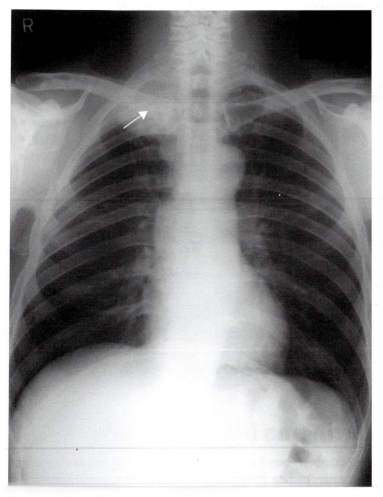

Fig. A22. PA chest radiograph showing normal heart size. In the right upper zone there is a soft tissue mass seen to be eroding the second rib (arrow). The hila appear normal. No other abnormality is seen in the lungs. The appearances are suspicious of a carcinoma of the bronchus involving the right lung apex which has eroded into the ribs. This is a Pancoast's tumour, also known as a superior sulcus tumour being essentially a tumour of the apex of the lungs. It can involve the cervical sympathetic chain and cause Horner's syndrome. It can also involve the brachial plexus (the T1 roots) and cause wasting of the interossei muscles of the hands.

This patient presented with fever, night sweats and weight loss.

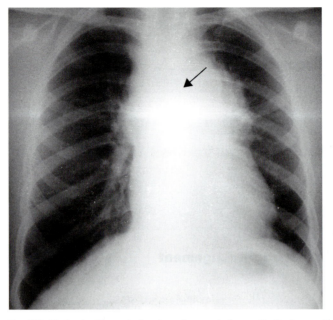

Fig. A32. PA chest radiograph showing a large anterior mediastinal mass. There is, in addition, bilateral hilar adenopathy. Note (arrow) how widened the anterior and superior mediastinum are compared with a normal chest radiograph. The lung parenchyma appear within normal limits. No pleural effusions are noted. Heart size is normal and no bony abnormalities are seen. The appearance in the context of the clinical history is likely due to nodes in the anterior mediastinum and the hilar regions in a patient with suspected lymphoma.

Mediastinal mass

The mediastinum is the space between the spine at the back, the sternum at the front and the lungs at the sides. It is divided into the anterior, middle and posterior mediastinum. Mediastinal lesions may cross from one compartment to another. Lesions in the mediastinum may be difficult to identify on a PA chest radiograph. A lateral film can be helpful but patients will usually need a CT scan of the chest to investigate suspected mediastinal lesions. The scan is performed with intravenous contrast that enhances the vessels in the mediastinum and enables them to be differentiated from other structures, e.g. nodes.

Anterior mediastinal masses

- Thyroid
- Thymus
- Teratoma
- Lymphoma

Middle mediastinal mass

- Lymphadenopathy
- Aortic aneurysm
- Hiatus hernia

Posterior mediastinal mass

- Neurogenic tumours, e.g. neurofibroma
- Aneurysm
- Paravertebral masses due to infection/tumour

This life-long smoker presented with clubbing and severe shortness of breath.

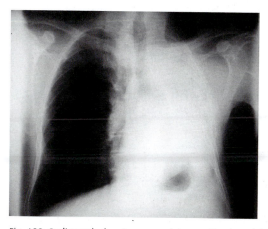

Fig. A33. Radiograph showing a complete opacification of the left hemi-thorax with mediastinal shift to the left. These are the signs of complete collapse of the left lung almost certainly due to a tumour, which was confirmed on bronchoscopy.

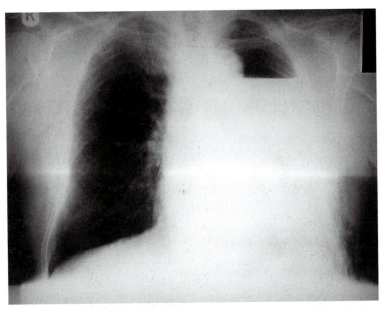

Fig. A34. Radiograph showing opacification of the left hemi-thorax with a fluid level present. There is also a little air seen in the soft tissues of the chest laterally (surgical emphysema). This patient has had a left pneumonectomy.

Opaque hemi-thorax

When faced with a chest radiograph showing a complete opacification of a hemi-thorax, check the trachea and the mediastinum to see if there is mediastinal shift present.

Causes of opaque hemi-thorax with shift away from the abnormal side

- Large pleural effusion

Central mediastinum

- Extensive consolidation

Mediastinal shift towards opaque side

- Collapse of lung secondary to obstructing tumour (usually central)
- Mucus plug (central) – especially post-operatively in intensive therapy unit (ITU), etc.

- Post-pneumonectomy – initially there will be a rising flood level until complete opacification occurs. Look for surgical emphysema (post-operative), rib resections

This patient presented with progressive shortness of breath. On examination he was clubbed and had basal inspiratory crackles on auscultation.

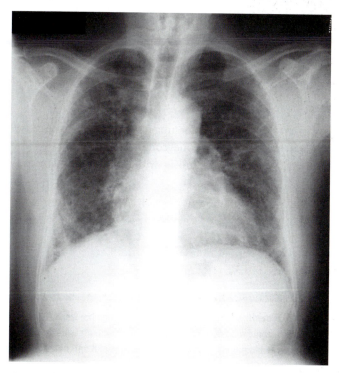

Fig. A35. Chest radiograph showing a fine reticulonodular shadowing in the bases which is making the lung bases a little indistinct. The lung volumes are still preserved. The appearances are seen in fibrosing alveolitis.

Cystic fibrosis

Cystic fibrosis is an autosomal recessive inherited disease in which there is an increased secretion of visceral mucus. In the lungs, small airways become obstructed with associated secondary infection.

Radiological signs in chest

- Thickening of bronchial walls (tram line)
- Bronchiectasis
- Patchy consolidation often in the upper/mid-zones
- Segmental collapse
- Mucus filled bronchi
- Focal emphysema/honeycombing
- Right-sided cardiac failure/pulmonary hypertension

Other features

- Abdomen
  - meconium ileus
  - dilated small bowel with thickened mucosal folds
  - pancreatic calcification
- Skeleton – retarded growth
- Sinuses
  - sinusitis
  - nasal polyps

A 40-year-old male patient presented with a chronic cough and repeated episodes of chest infection. Chest radiograph was unremarkable. What is this test and what does it show?

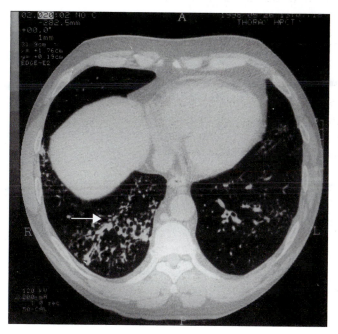

Fig. A39. Section of a high-resolution CT scan study of the chest. The technique takes thin sections of the chest allowing a very detailed look at the lung parenchyma. Bilateral basal bronchiectasis is seen (dilated bronchi in the periphery of the lung) (arrow).

Bronchiectasis

Bronchiectasis is the irreversible dilatation of the bronchi. It presents with recurrent cough and chest infections.

Radiological features

- Dilated bronchi
- Bronchial wall thickening
- Cystic spaces
- Associated emphysema

- Consolidation
- Fibrosis
- Chest radiograph may be normal in mild cases

Signs on CT scan (high resolution)

- Dilated bronchi
- Visible bronchi in periphery of lung
- Bronchial wall thickening
- Consolidated lung

Causes

- Childhood infections, e.g. measles, whooping cough
- Cystic fibrosis
- Congenital causes, e.g. Kartagener's syndrome (bronchiectasis, sinusitis, dextrocardia)
- Obstruction by foreign body, tumour
- Tuberculosis
  - usually bronchiectasis in upper lobes
  - bronchopulmonary aspergillosis

Pulmonary emboli

The patient presented with shortness of breath a week following surgery. What is the test and what does it show?

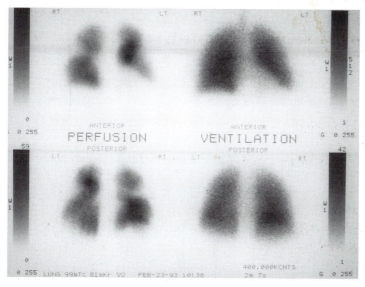

Fig. A40. VQ scan. This is a radioisotope investigation. The lung perfusion scan is performed with ^{99m}Tc macro-aggregated albumin, which is injected intravenously. This shows perfusion defects that correspond to pulmonary infarcts. The ventilation scan is performed using ^{81m}Kr, which the patient inhales.

These scans show a ventilation/perfusion (VQ) mismatch, which is a feature of pulmonary emboli.

Further investigations

- Spiral/multislice CT of the chest (CT pulmonary angiogram) can identify thrombi in the proximal pulmonary arteries (non-invasive test)
- Pulmonary angiogram – used to be considered 'Gold Standard' for the detection of pulmonary emboli but is invasive and is not routinely performed now
- Look for deep vein thrombosis in the legs using compression Doppler sonography

Chest X-ray for signs in pulmonary emboli

- Normal – commonest
- Wedge-shaped peripheral consolidation
- Pulmonary oligaemia
- Linear atelectasis
- Pleural effusion

Causes of matched perfusion defects on a VQ scan

- Pneumonia
- Pulmonary oedema
- COAD

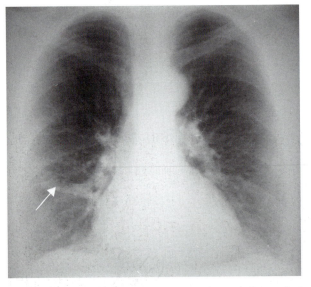

Fig. A41. Chest radiograph showing an area of linear atelectasis (collapse) in the right lung base in a patient with pulmonary embolus (arrow).

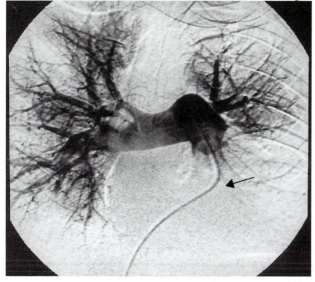

Fig. A42. Pulmonary angiogram showing no flow in the pulmonary arteries in the left lung base (arrow). The patient had an embolus blocking the region. The catheter tip is in the left pulmonary artery.

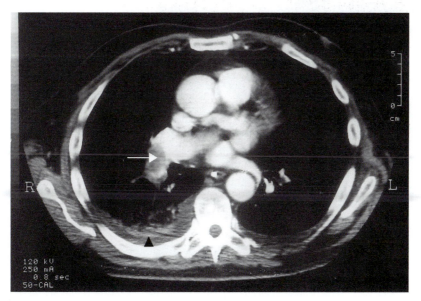

Fig. A43. Section of a spiral CT scan of the chest in another patient showing a filling defect in the right pulmonary artery (dark area) (arrow). There is also a small right pleural effusion (arrowhead).

ITU chest X-ray

On ITU the chest X-ray is taken supine and is an AP film. This can magnify the heart size. In addition pleural effusions do not show the meniscus sign but can appear as a generalized haziness on the film. Look out for the following lines or tubes:

- ECG leads
- Central lines – these are inserted through the jugular vein or the subclavian vein and the tip should be in the superior vena cava (SVC)
- Endotracheal tube – this lies in the trachea and the tip should be 5–7 cm from the carina
- Swan–Ganz catheter – this is introduced through the jugular vein and passed through the right atrium, right ventricle and into the pulmanry arteries where the tip of the catheter can be wedged to give a reading of the the left atrial pressure
- Pacemaker – the tip of the lead lies in the right ventricle
- Nasogastric tube – the tip should pass through the oesophagus into the stomach.

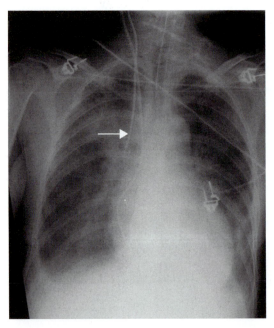

Fig. A44. Chest radiograph taken on an ITU patient showing an endotracheal tube *in situ*. The tip of the jugular line is in the SVC (arrow). There is a Swan–Ganz catheter in place to measure the pulmonary artery wedge pressure. In addition there is a right-sided pleural effusion seen with haziness extending into the right hemi-thorax which is a feature of the supine effusion. Also the ECG leads for cardiac monitoring.

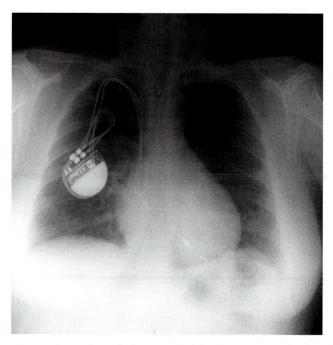

Fig. A45. Chest radiograph showing a dual chamber pacemaker. The tip of the wires are in the right atrium and the right ventricle.

Gastrointestinal system

Interpreting the abdominal radiograph

How the radiograph is taken

- A supine film is performed
- An erect chest radiograph is also helpful in identifying gas under the diaphragm in cases of perforation

Look for

- Name and markers
- Small bowel for obstruction (situated centrally with a diameter of <2.5 cm). Valvulae conniventes may be seen. Fluid may be seen in normal people
- Large bowel (peripherally placed). Haustra present. Calibre may be up to 10 cm
- Caecum >9 cm in large bowel obstruction. May lead to perforation
- Renal outline
- Calcification
  - renal
  - pancreatic
  - vascular
  - uterus
  - gallstones
  - bladder
- Unusual pockets of gas that do not lie in bowel (signifies perforation/abscess)
- Gas in biliary tree
- Hernial orifice (look for bowel as this might provide clue regarding hernia)
- Bony structures including lumbar spine and pelvis for degenerative disease, metastases

The following patient presented with a clinical history of severe central abdominal pain. On examination, generalized tenderness was noted. The patient underwent the following investigation.

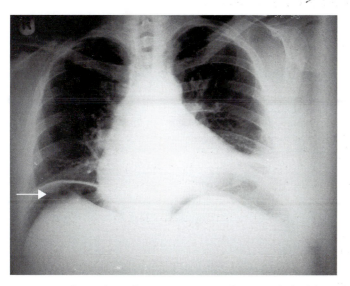

Fig. B1. Erect chest radiograph. Free intra-peritoneal gas is under both hemi-diaphragms. This is most noticeable under the right diaphragm where air is seen between the dome of the liver and the diaphragm (arrow). On the left side free intra-peritoneal air can sometimes be difficult to identify as there are often bowel loops present and a stomach bubble present at this site. These are the signs of a perforation in this clinical context. It is important that the patient is sat upright for at least 5–10 min to allow the intra-peritoneal air to appear under the diaphragms. If the patient cannot do this, perforation can be diagnosed on a plain abdominal film by looking for air on both sides of the bowel wall (Rigler's sign).

Perforation

Free gas outside the bowel lumen is an abnormal finding. Free intra-peritoneal gas is best seen on an erect chest radiograph as air under the right hemi-diaphragm. It is usually due to a perforation.

Causes of intra-peritoneal gas

- Following laparotomy/laparoscopy (air usually absorbed within 1 week)
- Colonic perforation, e.g. diverticular abscess, perforated duodenal ulcer

If there is doubt about a pneumoperitoneum, a left lateral decubitus film will demonstrate air in the flank.

Other causes of gas outside the bowel lumen

- Gas in an abscess (small bubbles of air may be seen)
- Gas in the bowel wall – seen in infarcted bowel
- May be benign (blobs of air seen in pneumatosis coli)
- Gas may be seen in the biliary system due to:
  - endoscopic retrograde cholangio-pancreatography (ERCP) + sphincterotomy
  - biliary operation
  - biliary fistula

This patient presented with abdominal distension following recent surgery. He underwent the following investigation.

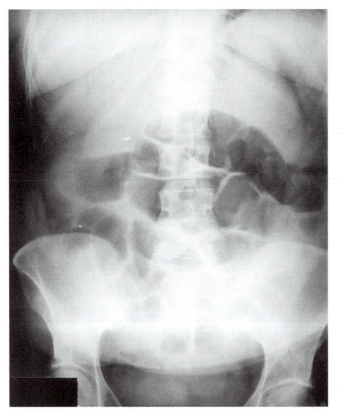

Fig. B2. Supine abdominal radiograph showing dilated loops of bowel situated centrally in the abdomen. Surgical clips are noted from a presumed cholecystectomy. The clips are identified in the right upper outer quadrant. This film does not include the hernial orifices. It is important that the hernial orifices are included on a film as this may demonstrate bowel in the hernia.

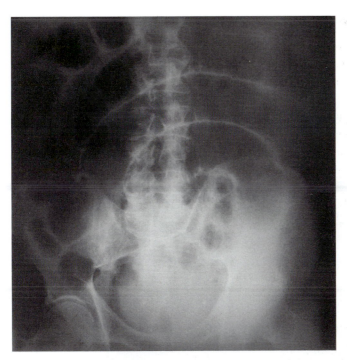

Fig. B3. Supine film also showing a dilated small bowel.

Small bowel obstruction

Signs of small bowel obstruction

- Dilated bowel loops are usually centrally placed in abdomen
- Several layered dilated loops often seen
- If the jejenum is dilated, the 'valvulae conniventes' may be seen crossing the width of bowel (stack of coins sign)
- Erect film not usually necessary as air/fluid levels in small bowel may be misleading

Causes of small bowel obstruction

- Adhesions
- Strangulated hernia
- Gallstone ileus
- Part of paralytic ileus
- Jejenum dilated if diameter >3.5 cm
- Ileum dilated if diameter >3 cm

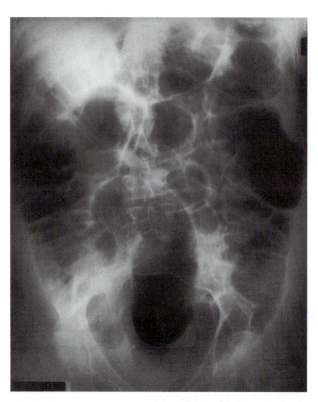

Fig. B4. The patient presented with slowly progressive distension of the abdomen. Plain abdominal radiograph showing dilated loops of bowel. The bowel, which is dilated, is seen in the peripheral distribution and extends from the ascending, to the transverse, to the descending colon. No clear cut-off is seen. The large bowel identified peripherally shows evidence of haustrae. No thickening of the bowel wall is demonstrated and there is no significant narrowing seen in any particular region.

Large bowel obstruction

Large bowel obstruction is usually seen secondary to an obstructing colonic carcinoma.

Abdominal film signs

- Large bowel is usually situated peripherally (cf. small bowel obstruction causes central dilated loops)
- Look for haustra of large bowel (cf. valvulae conniventes of small bowel)
- If ileocaecal valve is competent, caecal dilatation may be present. If caecum >9 cm there is a risk of perforation/infarction

- If ileocaecal valve is incompetent, accompanying small bowel obstruction may be present
- Look for collapsed bowel distal to obstruction

Causes

- Obstructing colonic carcinoma
- Diverticular disease
- Inflammatory bowel disease, e.g. Crohn's disease
- Infection, e.g. tuberculosis
- Volvulus of sigmoid colon
- Extrinsic compression by pelvic masses
- Hernia – usually causes small bowel obstruction
- Pseudo-obstruction – progressive dilatation of bowel seen in myxoedoema, post-pneumonia, myocardial infarction and medications
- Paralytic ileus – causes small and large bowel obstruction, especially in the post-operative stage

Further investigations

- Barium enema
- Abdomenal computed tomography (CT) to look for extrinsic cause

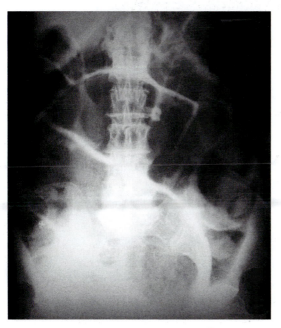

Fig. B5. Abdominal film showing a sigmoid volvulus with a dilated large bowel with inferior convergence to the left.

Signs of sigmoid volvulus

- Inferior convergence to the left
- Apex above T10 and under left hemi-diaphragm
- A haustral margin overlaps lower portion of liver
- Dilated descending colon in left side of pelvis

The patient presented with difficulty in swallowing. The following investigation was performed.

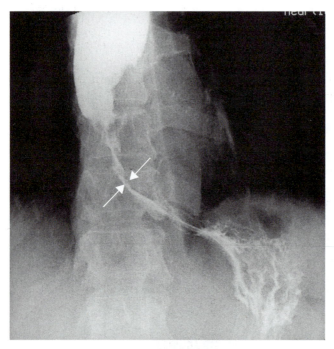

Fig. B6. A film taken from a barium swallow study demonstrating the region of distal oesophagus that is narrowed and irregular (arrows). There is some dilatation of the oesophagus proximal to this obstruction. There is little filling of the gastric fundus. The marked irregularity and narrowing seen in the distal oesophagus is almost certainly due to a carcinoma at this site.

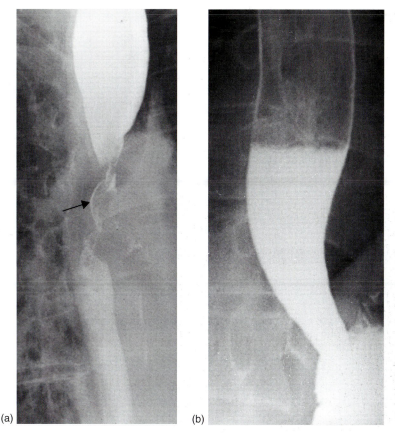

(a)   (b)

Fig. B7. (a) This film from a barium swallow showed narrowing in the mid-third of the oesophagus (arrow). (b) This film showed normal distal oesophagus on a barium swallow.

Barium swallow

On a normal barium swallow the oesophagus should have a smooth outline. No persistently narrowed areas should be seen. Peristalsis can be observed on screening the patient. The whole examination can be recorded on video if necessary (video-swallow examination).

Abnormalities

- Benign – stricture
  - reflux – stricture at lower end, short and smooth
  - corrosives – long stricture
- Achalasia – narrowing is seen in the distal oesophagus due to impaired relaxation of the lower oesophageal sphincter. Abnormal peristaltic activity is seen

- Malignant carcinoma – irregular narrowed lumen of oesophagus with 'shouldering'

Further investigations

- Endoscopy (enables biopsy)
- CT scan of thorax/abdomen to stage tumour, look for invasion of adjacent structures, nodes and metastases

Barium meals

The patient presented with heartburn, especially when bending over. This investigation was performed.

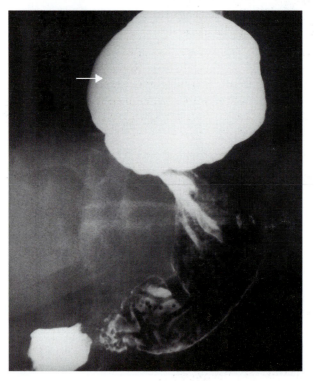

Fig. B8. Single film from a barium meal study. The stomach can be identified with the lesser curve and the greater curve seen quite clearly. This is a double-contrast examination, which means that the patient has been given a substance to produce gas inside the stomach such that adequate coating of the stomach can be performed and the stomach distended. A large barium-filled fundus is identified which lies above the level of the diaphragms. This is a hiatus hernia (arrow). A normal duodenal cap, which is also filled with barium, is identified.

The patient presented with epigastric pain, which was waking him at night. He underwent the following investigation.

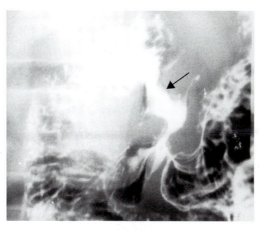

Fig. B9. Film taken from a barium meal study that shows the region of the duodenal cap (first part of the duodenum). This is abnormal and scarred and shows the presence of an ulcerated duodenal cap (arrow). Duodenal ulcers are now more often diagnosed using endoscopy rather than barium investigations. Complications of duodenal ulcers include perforation. If they perforate on the anterior surface, peritonitis may result. If they perforate through the posterior surface of the duodenum, penetration into the arteries may occur and the patient may present with a haematemesis.

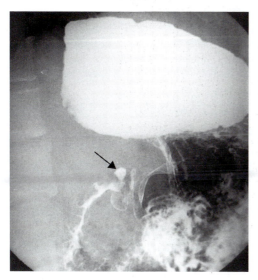

Fig. B10. Barium meal showing a pool of barium in the ulcer crater in the first part of the duodenum (arrow).

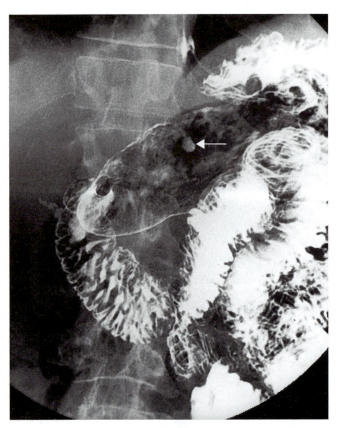

Fig. B11. Another film taken from a barium meal study. A pool of barium is seen on the posterior surface of the stomach wall (which is arrowed). This is an ulcer crater in the stomach. Whereas duodenal ulcers are nearly always benign, gastric ulcers have a potential for being malignant. An endoscopy is necessary to confirm the nature of this ulcer.

The patient presented with a change in bowel habit. He underwent the following investigation.

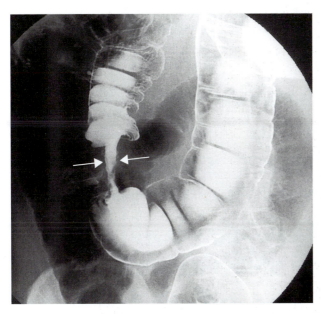

Fig. B12. Double-contrast barium enema. Barium has been introduced per rectum and passed round into the bowel. The next stage involves letting the barium out of the bowel and then introducing air to get sufficient distension to outline the mucosa of the bowel in detail. A narrowing is shown in the transverse colon (arrows). Barium passes through the narrowing and an irregularity is noted in the regions proximal and distal to the narrowed segment. This narrowed segment has the appearance of an apple core and is characteristic of a carcinoma of the bowel.

Bowel carcinoma

A normal barium enema will demonstrate the large bowel from the caecum on the right, the ascending, transverse and descending colon, and the sigmoid colon and rectum. Haustra may be seen (though not always present) and the bowel outline is smooth.

Features of bowel cancer on barium enema

- Narrowed segment 'apple core' lesion. This is due to the tumour growing around the bowel wall causing a narrowed irregular lumen

- Polypoid mass protruding into the lumen from the mucosal surface
- Plaque-like elevated growth from the mucosal surface (easily missed)

Causes of stricture on barium enema

- Diverticular disease
- Crohn's disease
- Ischaemic colitis
- Radiation fibrosis
- Infections, e.g. tuberculosis, amoebiasis

Further investigations

- Colonoscopy
- CT scan of the abdomen. This can also reveal bowel tumours and is helpful in staging
- CT Colonography can help identify polyps

The patient presented with intermittent left-sided abdominal pain. There was no history of anaemia or weight loss.

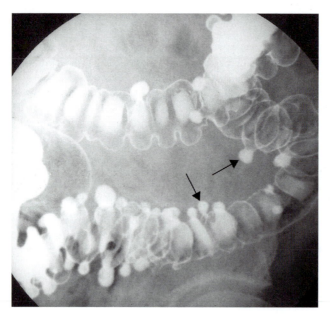

Fig. B13. Section of a sigmoid colon taken from a double-contrast barium enema study. The colon shows 'outpouchings' or diverticulae. No perforation or stricture seen (arrows).

Diverticular disease

Diverticular disease is common in the Western world due to the predominantly low fibre content in the diet. Diverticula are mucosal outpouchings through the muscular layer of the bowel wall. They are common in the sigmoid and descending colon. The patient may present with left iliac fossa pain.

Signs on barium enema

- Outpouchings may be filled with barium
- Diverticula seen outside bowel wall
- Fluid level may be present in diverticulum
- Diverticulae arise between mesenteric and anti-mesenteric taenia coli
- There may be associated muscle hypertrophy

Complications of diverticula

- Perforation and formation of diverticular peri-colic abscess (look for extravasation of barium)
- Fistula formation (look for barium track)
- Stricture in the bowel
- Haemorrhage

Remember

Polyps may be missed in the presence of diverticular disease

DO NOT FORGET CARCINOMA OF BOWEL MAY LOOK SIMILAR TO DIVERTICULAR STRICTURE

The patient presented with a history of diarrhoea. He underwent the following investigation.

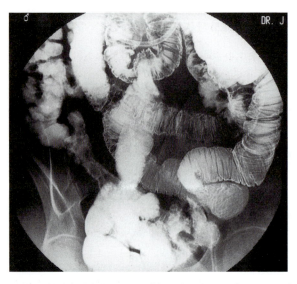

Fig. B14. Radiograph from a small bowel enema study. An irregular and narrowed terminal ileum is identified. The walls of the terminal ileum show evidence of rose thorn ulceration. A further more proximal area of abnormal mucosa is noted in the small bowel. This patient has the radiological signs on a barium study of Crohn's disease.

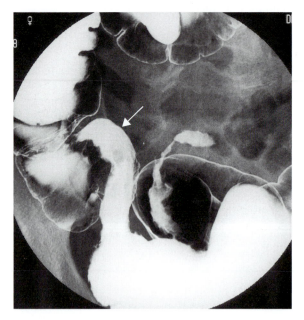

Fig. B15. Barium enema study showing that the barium has been refluxed through the ileocaecal valve into the terminal ileum. A narrowed irregular mucosal outline to the terminal ileum is also shown, which confirms the presence of Crohn's disease (arrow). This is another way of looking at the terminal ileum in patients with suspected Crohn's disease.

Crohn's disease

Crohn's disease is caused by a localized granulomatous inflammation that can affect any part of the gastrointestinal tract from the mouth to the anus. The exact cause is still unknown. The terminal ileum is the commonest site of involvement. Several areas of the bowel may be involved 'skip' lesions with normal bowel in between.

Investigations

- Plain abdominal film
- Barium follow through (patient drinks dilute barium and the barium is followed around the small bowel) – no intubation required, but it is not very accurate at detecting mucosal detail
- Small bowel enema – patient swallows a special nasogastric tube that is passed beyond the fourth part of the duodenum. Contrast is infused and spot films taken. Excellent mucosal detail obtained
- Barium enema – if colonic Crohn's disease is suspected

Signs on plain film

- Mucosal thickening
- Strictures with dilated bowel loops
- Gallstones
- Associated sacro-ileitis

Signs on small bowel enema

- Deep ulceration (rose thorn) in bowel wall
- Cobblestone mucosa (due to oedema)
- Stricture – solitary or multiple
- Terminal ileum fibrosis, stricture, spasm (string sign of Kantor)
- Thickening of valvulae conniventes
- Separation of bowel loops

Complications

- Bowel obstruction
- Fistula formation – to bowel, bladder and rectum
- Perforation/abscess formation
- Peri-anal involvement

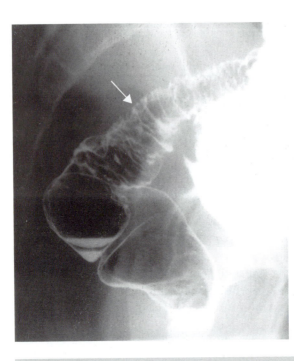

Fig. B16. Lateral rectum view of a barium enema showing a narrowed irregular sigmoid colon with rose thorn ulceration (arrow). This was due to Crohn's disease in the large bowel.

The patient presented with a history of bloody diarrhoea with mucus in the stools.

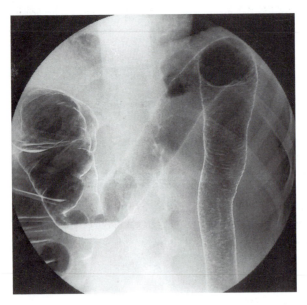

Fig. B17. Barium enema study showing a granular mucosal outline in the descending colon with loss of haustral folds. The diameter of the colon is within normal limits.

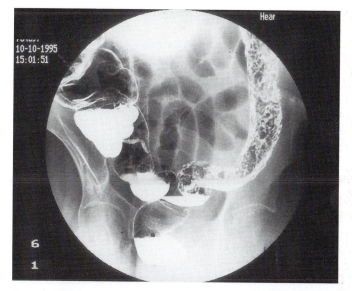

Fig. B18. Barium enema showing pseudopolyps in the descending colon.

Ulcerative colitis

Ulcerative colitis is characterized by inflammation and ulceration of the colon (aetiology unknown) with the patient presenting with bloody diarrhoea and mucus in stools. The rectum is always involved. When extensive, the whole colon may be affected (pancolitis).

Radiological signs

- Plain films of abdomen – mucosal thickening
- Dilated bowel (toxic megacolon) – a serious complication with risk of perforation
- Barium enema – mucosal granularity
- Mucosal oedema 'thumb printing'
- Loss of haustral folds
- Narrowed colon
- Pseudopolyps (10%) – swollen mucosa between ulcerated areas

Ulcerative colitis can be difficult to distinguish from Crohn's colitis (strictures are commoner in the latter).

Complications

- Toxic megacolon
- Carcinoma of colon commoner in long standing ulcerative colitis

Other causes of colitis

- Infective, e.g. amoebic, campylobacter, cytomegalovirus
- Ischaemic
- Radiation induced (following radiotherapy)

The patient presented with right upper abdominal discomfort. He underwent the following investigation.

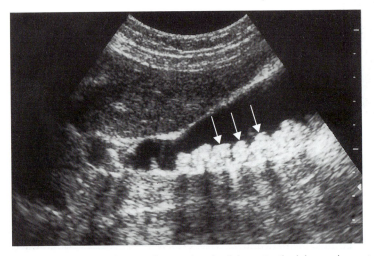

Fig. B19. Section taken from an ultrasound study of the patient's abdomen demonstrating a gallbladder (which appears black). Within the gallbladder on the posterior wall are multiple echogenic areas, which are gallstones (see arrows). Note the posterior acoustic shadowing (the black areas) characteristic of gallstones. On this particular section there is no evidence of a dilated intra-hepatic biliary system.

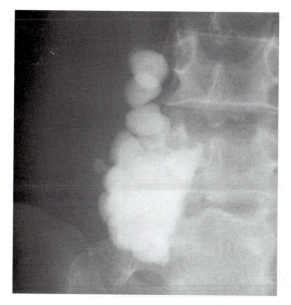

Fig. B20. Plain radiograph showing several stones in the gallbladder.

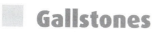 # Gallstones

Ultrasound is the first line investigation in patients with suspected gallstones. Ultrasound is non-invasive and uses the principles of reflected sound waves to create an image. It is a real-time investigation. Gallstones cause strong echogenic foci in the gallbladder (which appears black). In addition, acoustic shadows are seen behind the stones.

Causes of obstructive jaundice

- Gallstones in common bile duct
- Carcinoma of pancreas
- Tumour in porta hepatis

Investigation of obstructive jaundice

- Ultrasound – identifies gallstones, dilated biliary duct system and pancreatic tumours
- ERCP – visualizes the pancreatic ducts and the biliary duct system
- CT scan abdomen – identifies pancreatic tumours and spread. Dilated biliary system can also be seen

Liver metastases

The commonest tumour in the liver are secondary deposits from other tumours. Common tumours that metastasize to the liver are as follows:

- Lung
- Breast
- Colon
- Stomach
- Pancreas

Clinical presentation

- Weight loss
- Jaundice
- Hepatomegaly
- Abnormal liver function tests

Investigations

- Ultrasound – metastases are usually hypoechoic. However, the echo pattern of metastases are variable. Ultrasound contrast agents (intravenous) may help characterize lesions. Ascites can also be demonstrated as hypoechoic fluid in the abdomen
- CT scan – a multislice CT scan shows the arterial phase and the portal venous phase and can demonstrate abnormal regions in the liver
- Magnetic resonance imaging (MRI) – can be useful for demonstrating tumours
- Biopsy of lesions can be done under CT/ultrasound to obtain histology of the lesion

Liver metastases may be accompanied by ascites. This can be well demonstrated on ultrasound or CT scan.

Causes of ascites

- Cirrhosis
- Metastatic liver disease
- Cardiac failure
- Renal failure
- Tuberculous peritonitis
- Ovarian carcinoma

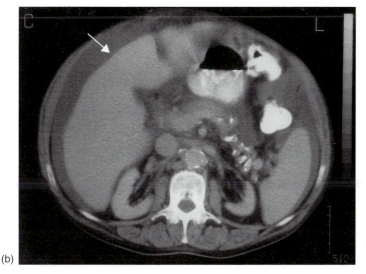

Fig. B29b. CT scan showing ascitic fluid around the liver (see arow).

Abdominal abscess

The patient presented with a temperature and a white count following recent abdominal operation.

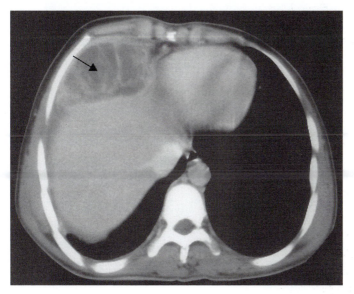

Fig. B30. Section of a CT scan at the level of the patient's upper abdomen showing an abnormal fluid collection between the liver and diaphragm. This is the site of a subphrenic abscess (arrow).

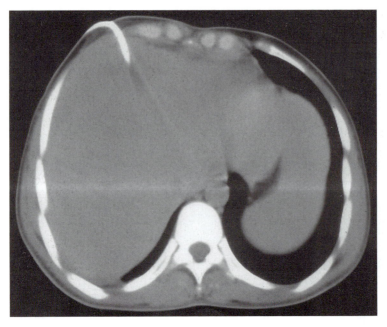

Fig. B31. CT section showing the presence of a drain within the abscess cavity that has been placed under radiological guidance.

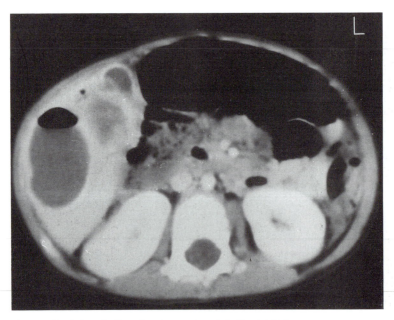

Fig. B32. CT section of a liver showing an abscess in the right lobe.

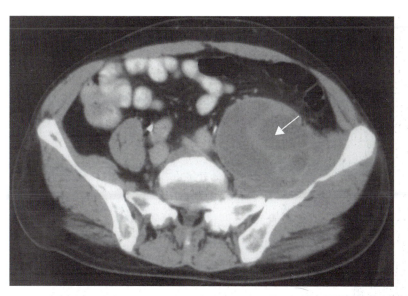

Fig. B33. CT scan of the lower abdomen showing a left psoas abscess (arrow).

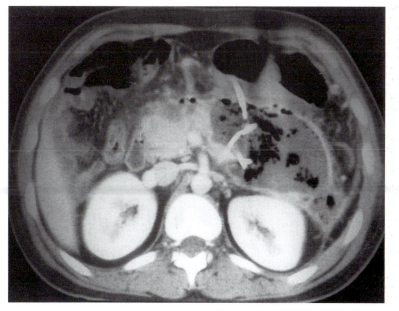

Fig. B34. CT scan of a pancreatic abscess (pockets of gas appear black) with a drain *in situ*.

Subphrenic abscess

Subphrenic abscess is an abnormal infected fluid collection between the diaphragm and liver or diaphragm and spleen.

Causes

- Following abdominal surgery
- Perforation

Investigations

- Chest X-ray – elevation of the diaphragm
- Ultrasound – demonstrates collection under the diaphragm
- CT scan – also demonstrates collections and enables the radiological drainage of the abscess under image guidance using catheters

Other sites of abscesses in abdomen (Figs B32–B34)

- Liver
  - pyogenic
  - amoebic
  - hydatid
- Renal
  - within kidney
  - perinephric
- Pancreatic – following pancreatitis
- Pelvic
  - post-surgery
  - diverticular abscess
- Appendix – abscess due to sealed-off perforation
- Psoas – tuberculosis

The central nervous system

CNS haemorrhage
Subarachnoid haemorrhage
Cerebral infarction
Brain atrophy
Ring enhancing lesions
MRI of the pituitary
Multiple sclerosis
Cerebrovascular disease

The patient presented confused after falling on his head. On examination there were right-sided neurological signs present.

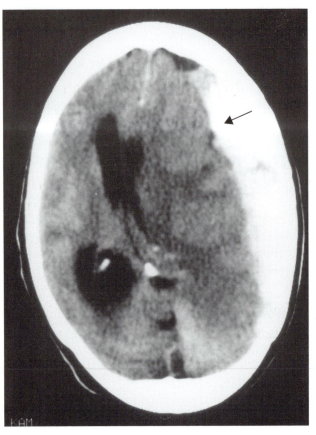

Fig. C1. Section of a CT scan of the brain. A high attenuation abnormal area is seen in the subdural space on the left side(see arrow). This is compressing the normal left cerebral hemisphere and is causing a mass effect such that there is compression of the left lateral ventricle and a shift of the midline to the right. These are the features of an acute subdural haematoma.

CNS haemorrhage

Head injuries are a common clinical problem especially in casualty departments. The investigation of choice in patients with neurological signs is a CT scan.

Although skull X-rays may show a fracture, they do not provide information about the brain parenchyma. In addition, there may be quite significant brain pathology in the absence of fractures on the skull radiograph.

The following may be seen following trauma:

Extra-dural haemorrhage

- Often due to ruptured middle meningeal artery
- CT scan shows a high attenuation (white) mass (fresh blood) peripherally around the brain adjacent to the cranial vault. The inner margin is often convex. Requires urgent neurological drainage

Subdural haemorrhage

- May present following a fall (often in alcoholics) with fluctuating consciousness. CT scan shows areas of crescentic peripheral high attenuation (white) with a concave inner border
- Midline shift may be seen to the opposite side of haemorrhage
- Mass effect may compress ventricles
- If subdural >2 weeks old, the blood may be hypodense (grey)

Intra-cerebral haemorrhage

- Focal area of increased attenuation (white) fresh blood
- May cause mass effect with midline shift
- Blood may extend into the ventricles

Also seen in haemorrhage due to:

- Hypertensive bleed (haemorrhagic stroke)
- Drugs, e.g. warfarin (over anticoagulation)
- Thrombocytopaenia
- Ruptured aneurysm

Cerebral contusion

- High attenuation areas in the brain are accompanied by brain swelling
- May be multi-focal
- Haemorrhage may be present in areas of contusion
- Due to shearing of white matter tracts, cerebral swelling may cause compression of ventricles and effacement of sulci

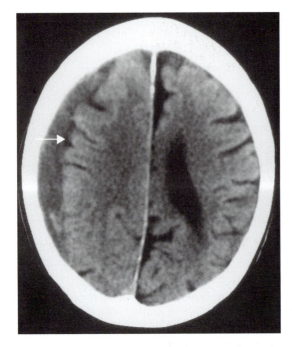

Fig. C2. CT scan showing low attenuation fluid collection around the right cerebral hemisphere (see arrow). Fluid collection is in the right subdural space and it is causing a minimal amount of mass effect. The appearances are those of a chronic right subdural haematoma. The right lateral ventricle is not clearly seen.

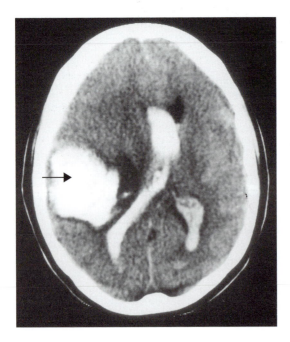

Fig. C3. Section of a CT scan showing a very large right-sided intra-cerebral haematoma (see arrow). The blood is fresh because the attenuation is white. Fresh bleeding causes a mass effect with a midline shift to the left side, away from the lesion. In addition, as seen, there is high attenuation (white) area in the lateral ventricles. This is due to the fact that there has been intra-ventricular haemorrhage.

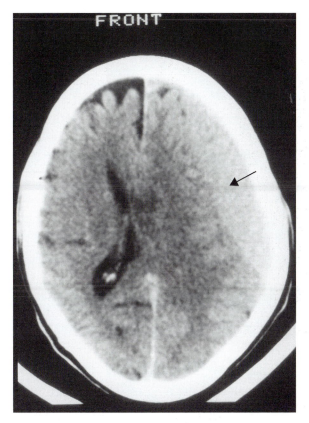

Fig. C4. CT scan of the brain. There is an abnormal area of isodense attenuation seen in the left subdural space (see arrow). This area is not white (i.e. it is not fresh blood). It is not of low attenuation either (i.e. it is not chronic). This density is almost similar to that of normal brain tissue. This is due to the fact that this haemorrhage is perhaps ~1 week old and is passing through the phase where the blood goes from appearing bright white to dark on the scan. These subdurals are easy to miss. Look very carefully for the mass effect. One can see that there is no left lateral ventricle clearly seen. In addition, one can see that the sulci are not clearly seen on the left side because there is a subdural collection at this site that is compressing the normal brain tissue.

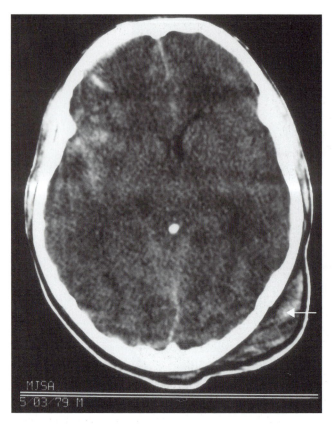

Fig. C5. CT scan of the brain. Note the soft tissue abnormality outside the left occipital bone (see arrow). This is a soft tissue haematoma in the superficial tissues of the skull at the back. The patient has been attacked and hit on the back of the head. There are patchy areas of increased attenuation (white) seen diagonally in the right frontal lobe that represent areas of contusion and haemorrhage at this site. This is called a contra-coup injury.

Subarachnoid haemorrhage

The patient presented with a sudden onset of headache.

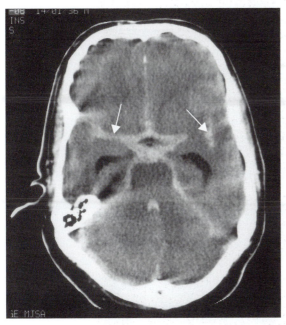

Fig. C6. CT scan of the brain and this section shows a marked high attenuation material in the cisterns of the brain and in the subarachnoid spaces. These are the appearances of a large subarachnoid haemorrhage.

Causes of subarachnoid haemorrhage

- Rupture of intra-cerebral aneurysm
- Arterio-venous malformation

Complications of subarachnoid

- Re-bleed
- Hydrocephalus (communicating)

Further tests

- Lumbar puncture (LP) – Remember 1–5% of subarachnoid haemorrhage may have a normal CT brain scan – hence importance of LP to look for xanthochromia.

- MR angiogram or CT angiogram – non-invasive
- Cerebral angiogram – invasive

Cerebral infarction

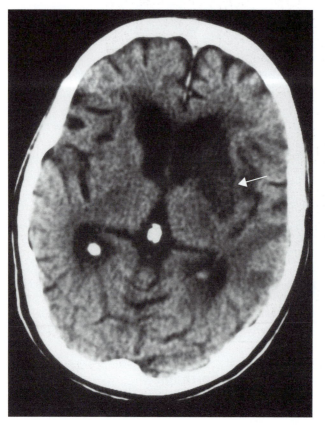

Fig. C7. CT scan of the brain showing a section at the level of the thalamus. There is a generalized atrophy noted. In addition, a low attenuation area is in the left side of the brain involving the left basal ganglia. This low attenuation region is not causing any significant mass effect. The appearances are those of an infarction of the left basal ganglia (see arrow).

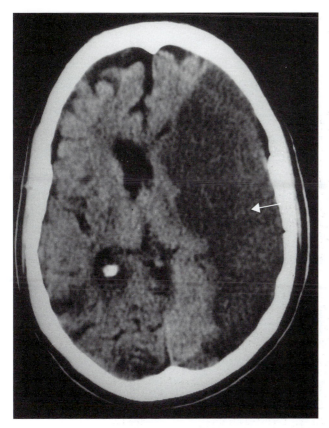

Fig. C8. CT section of the brain showing marked low attenuation in the left hemisphere with sparing of the left frontal lobe and left occipital lobe. These are the appearances of massive infarction of the left side of the brain due to an occlusion involving the left middle cerebral artery (see arrow).

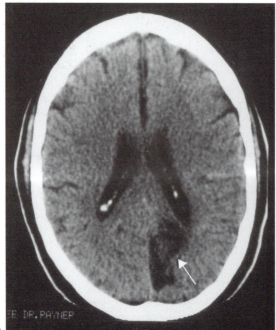

(a)

Fig. C9a. CT scan of the brain at the level of the occipital lobes showing a low attenuation (dark) area in the left occipital lobe (see arrow). This is due to an infarct involving the left posterior cerebral artery.

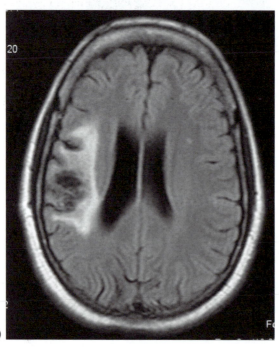

(b)

Fig. C9b. MRI scan of brain following intravenous contrast (gadolinium chelate) showing gyral enhancement in right hemisphere (white area) following an infarct. The enhancement of the gyrus is due to luxury perfusion which may be present at the site of an infarct.

Cerebral infarction

Cerebral infarction is due to an impaired circulation of the brain. A thrombus or an embolus causes it (often from the carotid vessels). The clinical presentation is that of a stroke.

Investigations

- CT scan – used to identify an infarct and to rule out a haemorrhage as the cause of a stroke. In the early stages (first 24 h) the scan may be normal in an infarct
  - early signs include loss of grey–white matter interface
  - a reduced density is noted in the brain, and the area involved usually corresponds to the arterial supply affected (e.g. anterior, middle or posterior cerebral artery territories)
  - luxury perfusion may be present
  - oedema and swelling in the early stages with mass effect
  - infarcts may be haemorrhagic
  - old infarcts show areas of low attenuation
- MRI scan
  - shows an area of increased signal on a T2-weighted image of the site of the infarct
  - posterior fossa and brain stem infarcts are better seen using MRI
- Carotid ultrasound – allows visualization of the common carotid and internal carotid arteries to look for plaque (soft or calcific) and narrowing of the vessels

Stroke (WHO definition) is the rapid onset of focal (global) cerebral deficit lasting more than 24 h or leading to death due to a vascular cause,

- Three types
- Ischaemic stroke 80%
- Intra-cerebral haemorrhage 15%
- Subarachnoid haemorrhage 5%

Brain atrophy

Brain atrophy is due to the irreversible loss of brain tissue. Atrophy of the brain occurs with ageing and in elderly patients it is common to see the loss of brain tissue.

Radiological signs on CT/MRI

- Increased cerebro-spinal fluid (CSF) space with widening of the sulci
- Prominent ventricles
- Prominent basal cisterns and temporal horns of lateral ventricles
- In Alzheimer's disease there may be cerebellar sparing

Causes of atrophy

- Ageing
- Alzheimer's disease
- AIDS
- Trauma – long-term sequelae
- Congenital diseases of the brain
- Alcohol abuse (chronic)
- Radiotherapy
- Degenerative diseases

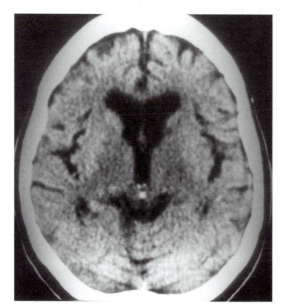

Fig. C10. CT scan of the brain showing features of atrophy. These include the prominent sulci and slightly dilated ventricles present in an atrophic brain.

This patient presented with a history of confusion following treatment of bronchial carcinoma.

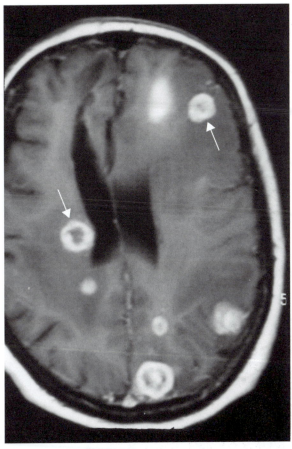

(a)

Fig. C11a. MRI scan of a section of the brain showing multiple ring enhancing regions in the brain (see arrow). Some are associated with oedema (dark grey area). This scan has been performed with intravenous contrast to demonstrate the ring enhancement of metastatic disease.

Ring enhancing lesions

Ring enhancing lesions identified on a MRI or CT scan are due to:

- Metastases
- Cerebral abscesses
- Primary brain tumour

On a CT scan the lesions may be associated with cerebral oedema identified by areas of lower density around the lesion. On an MRI scan, oedema appears as bright signal on T2-weighted images. The swelling may cause compression of the ventricles and midline shift.

Common primary tumours that metastasize to the brain

- Lung
- Breast
- Colon

Common abscesses

- Toxoplasma in patients with AIDS
- *Staphylococcus* due to:
  - blood-borne infection, e.g. endocarditis
  - direct from mastoiditis, sinusitis
- Tuberculosis

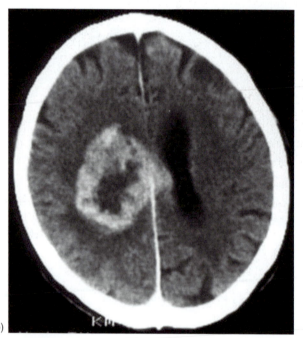

(b)

Fig. C11b. CT scan of brain following intravenous contrast showing an irregular enhancing mass in right hemisphere with features suggestive of a primary malignant brain tumour such as a glioma.

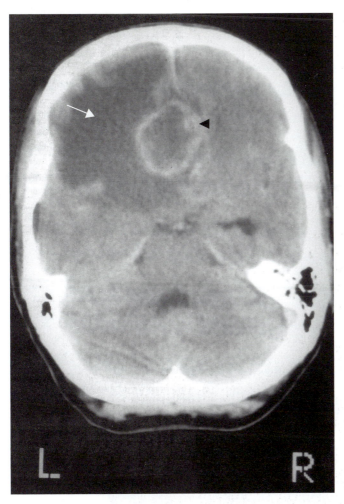

Fig. C12. Section of a brain scan in a patient with AIDS. It has been performed with intravenous contrast showing a ring enhancing abscess (see arrowhead), which in patients with AIDS is usually due to toxoplasmosis. The dark area around the abscess is due to oedema in the frontal lobe (see arrow). A repeat scan following treatment showed improvement in the abscess.

The patient presented with bi-temporal hemianopia.

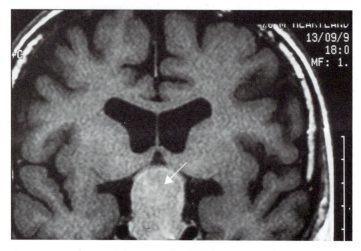

Fig. C13. Coronal section of a MRI study of the brain performed through the pituitary gland. A large mass is seen arising from the pituitary fossa. This is a mass arising from the pituitary gland and is, in fact, compressing on the optic chiasm. The mass is not involving the cavernous sinuses. It is not infiltrating into the temporal lobes. The appearances are those of an enlarging pituitary tumour involving the optic chiasm.

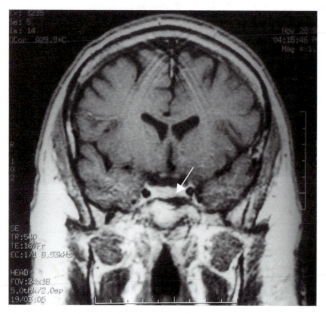

Fig. C14. Coronal section through a normal pituitary gland.

MRI of the pituitary

MRI is the radiological investigation of choice for patients with suspected pituitary tumours. Tumours may be either:

- Micro-adenomas (<1 cm)
- Macro-adenomas (>1 cm)
- When the tumour enlarges it grows out of the pituitary fossa
- Tumour may grow upwards and compress the optic chiasm (bi-temporal hemianopia)
- May be lateral spread into the cavernous sinuses (carotid artery and cranial nerve involvement)
- May be downward growth into the sphenoidal sinus

Pituitary tumours

- Secretory
- Prolactinomas (35%)
- Acromegaly (growth hormone) (25%)
- Cushings' (5%)
- Non-secretory (20%)

Differential diagnosis of pituitary tumours

- Craniopharyngioma
- Aneurysm
- Supra-sellar meningioma

A 25-year-old patient presented with a history of visual disturbances and pins and needles on two separate occasions.

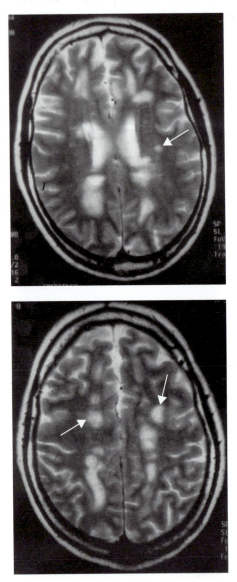

Figs. C15 (top) and 16 (bottom) Axial sections of an MRI study of the brain. This is in fact a T2-weighted sequence (the CSF and the ventricle appear white). There are areas of increased signal (white) in the white matter of the brain. These have the appearances of plaques of de-myelination and in someone of this age group a diagnosis of multiple sclerosis would be considered. In elderly patients these areas of increased signal (hyperintensities) are quite commonly seen and are often due to vascular changes in an elderly brain.

Multiple sclerosis

Multiple sclerosis is a disease predominantly of the young adult characterized by plaques of de-myelination in the brain and spinal cord. Relapse and remission characterize it, although it may show progression to chronic disability in a number of cases. Imaging has revolutionized the diagnosis of this disease although a detailed history and examination are of paramount importance, as imaging is not always specific.

CT findings

- Low attenuation areas in white matter
- Atrophy
- CT is **not** the first line imaging investigation of choice

MRI findings

- First-line imaging investigation
- Multiple high signal areas are seen in the brain on T2-weighted images
- High signal areas <2 cm
- High signal areas have smooth margins, are ovoid and are often periventricular in location
- High signal areas may be present in the spinal cord or optic nerves
- Active plaques may enhance with contrast
- The most sensitive MRI sequence for detecting lesions is the fluid attenuated inversion recovery (FLAIR) sequence

Differential diagnosis of white matter intensities on MRI

- Age-related changes
- Ischaemic changes
- Vasculitis
- HIV dementia

The patient presented with transient ischaemic attacks and underwent the following test.

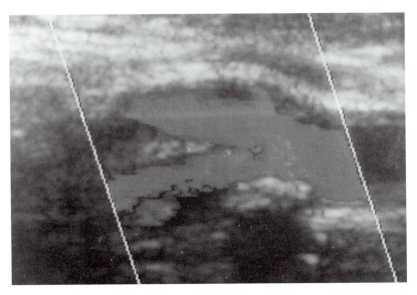

Fig. C17. Doppler investigation of the carotid artery. The section shows a calcified plaque at the origin of the internal carotid artery that appears to be causing some narrowing of the internal carotid artery. The plaque is causing some shadowing. This is the feature of a calcified plaque. The appearances are those of a plaque causing some narrowing of the internal carotid artery. Both the carotid bulb and the common carotid artery appear normal.

Cerebrovascular disease

Cerebrovascular disease is a major cause of morbidity and mortality in the Western world. Investigation of the carotid arteries may be helpful in identifying plaques and narrowing in the carotid bifurcation.

Until recently, investigation of the carotid bifurcation required invasive carotid angiography. Today, however, the first line investigation is a non-invasive carotid Doppler ultrasound investigation. Doppler ultrasound involves three steps:

- Inspection of the carotid vessels in a longitudinal plane on standard grey-scale images
- Colour Doppler to outline the stenoses
- Spectral Doppler to measure velocities of blood flow in vessels to enable quantification of stenoses

Doppler ultrasound can demonstrate.
- Narrowing
- Plaques
- Intimal thickening

Other radiological tests

- Magnetic resonance angiography
  - can identify the carotid bifurcation
  - stenoses overestimated
- Invasive carotid angiography – allows angioplasty of certain lesions (risk of stroke)

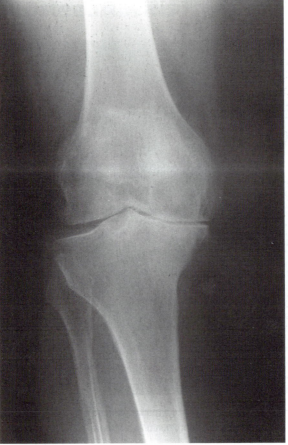

Fig. D3. Radiograph of a knee joint showing degenerative change in the medial compartments of the knee joint with loss of joint space when compared with the lateral compartment.

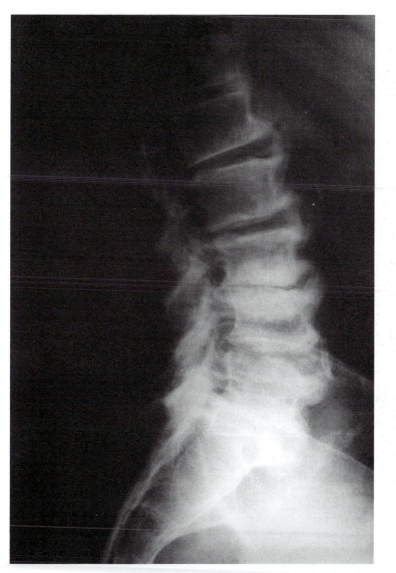

Fig. D4. Lateral radiograph of the lumbar spine showing degenerative change in the L3/4, L4/5 and L5/LS1 levels with loss of joint space, loss of disc height, sclerosis adjacent to the end-plates and anterior osteophytes at a number of levels.

The commonest form of arthritis is osteoarthritis. It is due to degenerative change in the articular cartilage of joints due to wear and tear. Osteoarthritis becomes frequent as one ages.

Radiological changes

- Loss of joint space, often greatest in weight-bearing joints. The joint space becomes narrowed
- Osteophyte formation – bony outgrowths seen at the articular margin of joints
- Subchondral sclerosis
- Subchondral cysts (geodes)
- Loose bodies – pieces of calcified cartilage in joint spaces

Common sites

- Cervical spine – narrowed disc space osteophytes, narrowed intervertebral foramane (Fig. D2)
- Lumbar spine – narrowed disc space, osteophytes (Fig. D4)
- Hip joints – loss of joint space, subchondral sclerosis, may be accompanied by femoral head deformity (Fig. D1)
- Knee – loss of joint space in medial compartment and patello-femoral compartments, loose bodies in joints (Fig. D3)
- Hands – distal interphalangeal joint, narrowing base of first metacarpal/ carpal joint

Rheumatoid arthritis

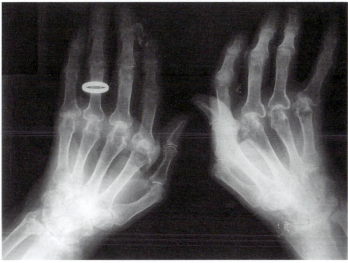

(a)

Fig. D5a. Radiographs of the hands of a patient with severe rheumatoid arthritis. Note the erosive changes in the metacarpal phalangeal joints, especially of the second, third and fourth digits. In addition, note the angulation deformity present at the joints and also the generalized osteopenia. An erosion is also noted in the distal ulna of the right hand. In the later stages there may be ankylosis of joints present.

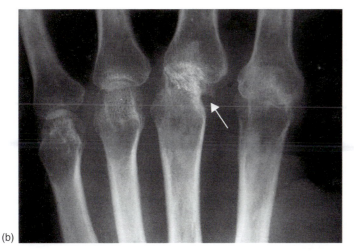

(b)

Fig. D5b. Radiograph showing an erosion in the head of the third metacarpal at the metacarpo-phalangeal joint (see arrow).

Gout

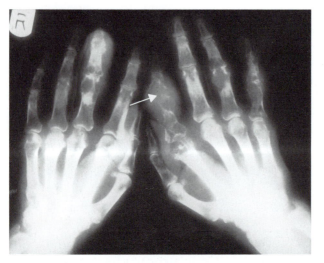

Fig. D6. Patient presenting with painful red, swollen joints in the hands and toes. A marked soft tissue swelling around the joints with erosive changes is shown. The appearances are seen in gouty arthritis due to raised uric acid levels (see arrow).

Radiology of gout

- Asymmetrical arthritis
- Predilection for metatarso-phalangeal joint of toe
- Soft tissue swelling (tophi) around joints
- Punched out juxta-articular erosions

Rheumatoid arthritis

Rheumatoid arthritis is a chronic polyarthritis in which synovial proliferation occurs leading to a chronic synovitis. Common joints affected include:
- Hands (Fig. D5)
- Feet
- Wrist
- Cervical spine
- Knees

Radiological findings

Early signs include:
- Soft tissue swelling
- Osteoporosis

- Joint space narrowing due to cartilage destruction
- Erosions at joint margins
  - metatarso-phalangeal joints
  - metacarpo-phalangeal joints
  - styloid process of ulna
- Disruption of joint surfaces leads to ulnar deviation in the wrists
- Subluxation at the MCP joints
- Eventual fusion of carpal bones
- Erosion of acromio-clavicular joints
- Atlanto-axial subluxation in the cervical spine
- Baker's cyst in the knee

Remember osteoarthritis may also be present. Radiology can be used to monitor progress of the disease.

Ankylosing spondylitis

A male patient presented with a progressively stiff back and neck.

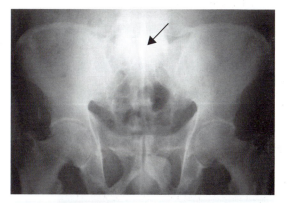

Fig. D7. Pelvic radiograph showing sclerosis and fusion of the sacro-iliac joints and calcification of the interspinous ligaments characteristic of ankylosing spondylitis (see arrow).

Radiology

- Sacroileitis
- Squaring of vertebra of spine
- Calcification of longitudinal ligaments, anterior and lateral spinal ligaments to produce a 'bamboo' spine
- Apical fibrosis on chest radiographs

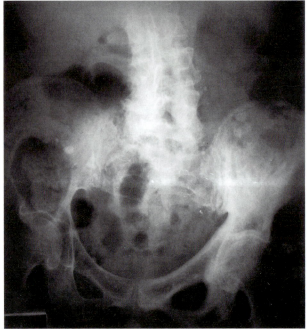

(a)

Fig. D8a. Plain abdominal radiograph showing a coarsened trabeculation in the left iliac bone and also a quite marked coarsened trabeculation and periosteal thickening involving the left superior pubic ramus and acetabulum, as well as the left inferior pubic ramus. These are the appearances of Paget's disease involving the left hemi-pelvis. In addition, there is some degenerative change in the left hip joint. The lumbar spine shows evidence of degenerative change with a scoliosis (curvature) convex to the left.

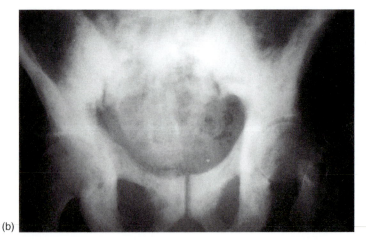

(b)

Fig. D8b. Pelvic radiograph showing sclerotic bone in the pubic rami, ischium and iliac bones. The bones are denser than normal.

Paget's disease

Paget's disease of bone is often an incidental finding.

Presentation

- Incidental finding
- Bone pain
- Fractures
- Bone deformity

Paget's disease can affect any bone, but the following are the commonest areas:

- Skull
  - well-defined area of bone loss (osteoporosis circumscripta)
  - sclerosis and expansion of the skull vault ('cotton wool')
  - enlargement of the head
  - otosclerosis
  - platybasia
- Pelvis – coarsening of trabeculae and sclerosis of ischium, pubis and ileum
- Femur/long bones
  - expansion and coarsening of trabeculae
  - expansion of cortex
  - bowing/deformity
- Spine – sclerosis of vertebrae

Complications

- Bone deformities
- Fractures
- Degenerative change
- Osteogenic sarcoma
- Cardiac failure

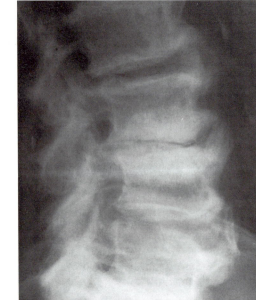

Fig. D9. Lateral radiograph of a lumbar spine showing loss of joint space between the vertebral bodies in the lower lumbar spine with sclerosis in the end plates. In addition, there is marked florid osteophyte formation noted in the anterior aspects of the vertebrae. The joint space at L5/S1 is also narrowed. These are the appearances of severe degenerative disease.

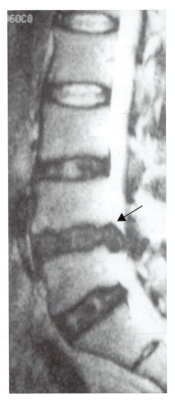

Fig. D10. Magnetic resonance imaging (MRI) scan of the lumbar spine. The section is taken from a T2-weighted sequence and the degenerative discs appear black; a posterior disc bulge is noted at the level of L4/L5. This is impinging on the roots and would account for the patient's symptoms (see arrow).

Back pain

Back pain is a common clinical problem and in most cases it does not require imaging. If neurological signs are present, however, urgent investigation may be necessary.

Common causes

- Acute disc prolapse
- Acute on chronic disc prolapse
- Metastases (in the elderly)
- Osteoporotic collapse
- Myeloma
- Infective discitis

Investigations

- Plain lumbar spine postero-anterior (PA) and lateral
  - may show collapse of vertebral body
  - may show loss of disc height/osteophytes
  - may show absent pedicles or destroyed vertebral bodies if metastatic disease is present
  - may show irregular end plates if infective discitis is present
  - may show pars interarticularis defect
- MRI lumbar spine
  - will demonstrate disc prolapse – commonest at L3/4 and L4/5 and L5/S1 levels and root compression if present
  - MRI is also more sensitive at detecting secondary deposits in the vertebral bodies

Myelography involves the injection of contrast medium into theca via lumbar puncture to demonstrate disc prolapse, etc. It is rarely performed now due to a wider availability of MRI scanning which is non-invasive.

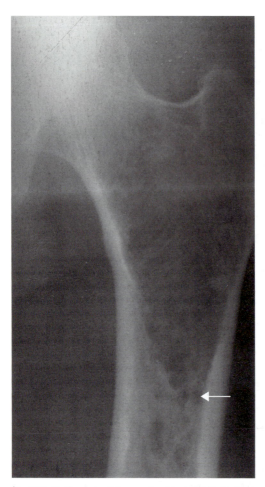

Fig. D12. Radiograph of the proximal femoral shaft. The bone is a little osteopenic. In the femoral shaft, however, lytic lucent areas are present. These are the appearances of myeloma deposits seen in a condition known as multiple myeloma. Remember that on a radio-isotope bone scan multiple myeloma may show cold spots, i.e. reduced uptake, compared with metastases which show increased uptake (see arrow).

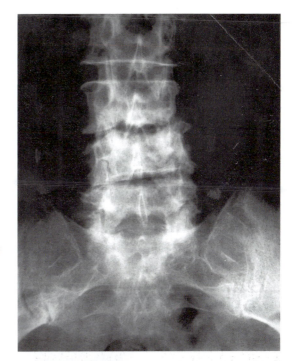

Fig. D13. Antero-posterior (AP) radiograph of a lumbar spine showing irregularity of the L4/5 lumbar vertebrae with loss of joint space and an irregular outline to the cortex. This is suspicious of an infection in the disc space causing a discitis.

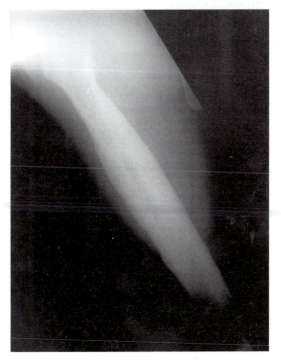

Fig. D14. Radiograph of a right femur showing marked periosteal reaction with marked thickening of the cortex and sclerosis of the cortical bone of the mid-shaft of the femur. In addition, the clear differentiation between the cortex and the medulla is lost in the mid-shaft. These are the appearances of a chronic osteomyelitis may be difficult to detect, as the only visible sign is a periosteal reaction that is not often seen until the disease is quite advanced.

Osteomyelitis

Osteomyelitis is an infection of the bone and is usually caused by *Staphylococcus aureus*. Chronic osteomyelitis may be caused by tuberculosis. Osteomyelitis presents with bone pain. It may be acute or chronic.

Radiological signs

- Acute osteomyelitis – no change seen in early osteomyelitis. On plain films signs include:
  - soft tissue swelling
  - periosteal reaction
  - bone destruction (earliest at metaphysis)
  - original bone may die forming separate isolated fragments (sequestrum)
- Chronic osteomyelitis (Fig. D14)
  - bone shows sclerotic reaction
  - loss of differentiation between cortex and medulla
  - sequestra may be seen within bone

Other investigations

- Radioisotope bone scans may show increased uptake
- MRI scans may show abnormal signal

Complications

- Fistula
- Abscess
- Deformity of joints

Remember that a bone tumour can be difficult to differentiate from osteomyelitis.

Metastases

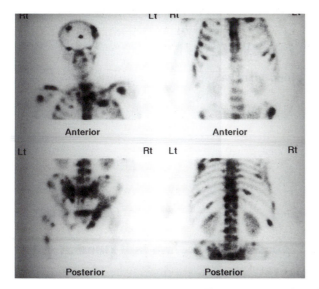

Fig. D15. Radio-isotope bone scan with (black) areas of increased uptake of isotope (so-called hot spots) throughout the skeleton. These are suspicious of metastases. It is important to remember that increased uptake can occur in fractures and also in degenerative disease.

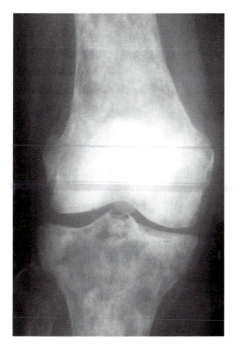

Fig. D16. Plain radiograph of the knee. A permeative destruction of bone is noted in the distal femur and proximal tibia. A marked lytic destruction is seen and these are the appearances of metastases.

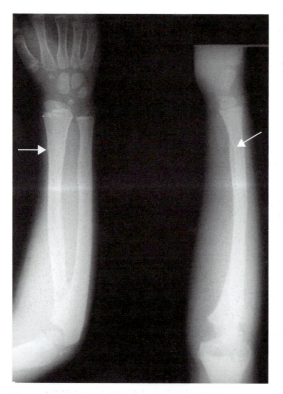

Fig. D27. Radiograph of the forearm of a child shown in two views. Note the buckling of the cortex in the distal radius due to a greenstick fracture (see arrows).

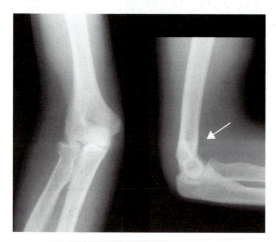

Fig. D28. Two views of elbow showing fracture of radial head and lateral view showing displaced anterior fat pad. Fat pads lie adjacent to the joint capsule and in the presence of an effusion following trauma in the joint the anterior and posterior fat pads are displaced (see arrow).

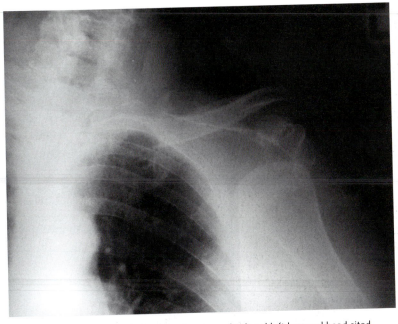

Fig. D29. Radiograph of a left shoulder showing a displaced left humeral head sited anteriorly. This is an example of an anterior dislocation of the left shoulder. These may be accompanied by an associated fracture.

Fig. D
over t
contir
(see a

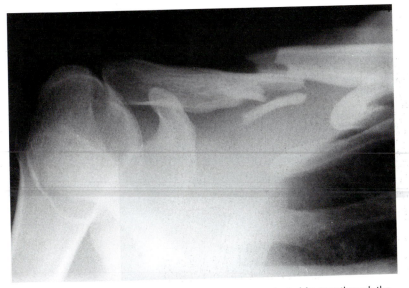

Fig. D30. Radiograph of the right shoulder showing a comminuted fracture through the mid-shaft of the right clavicle. Note that the fragment that is loose and separate from the clavicle. The bone is displaced.

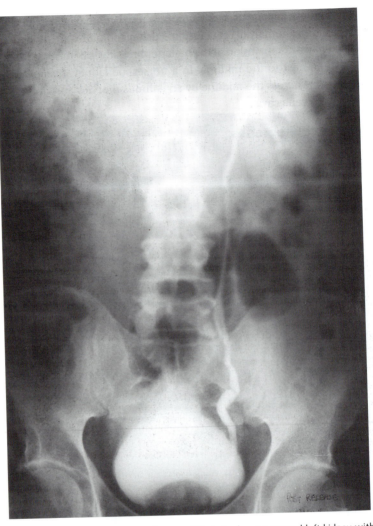

Fig. E3. A 15-min abdominal film from an IVP study shows a normal left kidney with an absent right kidney.

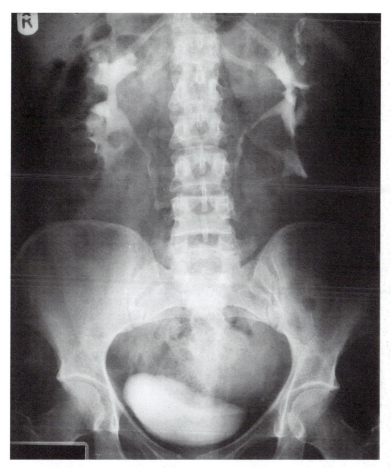

Fig. E4. A 15-min film from an IVP study showing bilateral enlarged kidneys with splayed calyces suggestive of polycystic kidneys. This can be confirmed on ultrasound by the identification of multiple cysts.

Renal colic

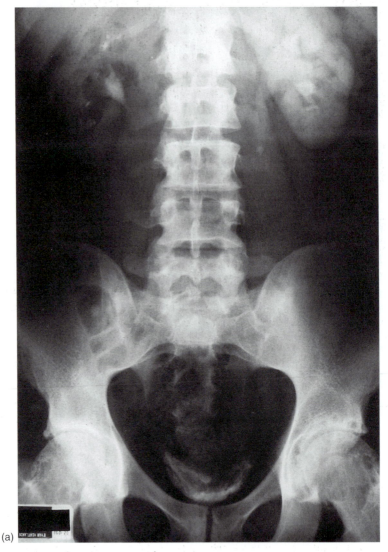

(a)

Fig. E5a. A patient presenting with colicky left-sided pain radiating from the left flank to the groin.

A 20-min film from an intravenous pyelogram (IVP) taken on a patient with left-sided renal colic. Note the dilated left collecting system that comes to a halt at the level of the left transverse process of L3 where the stone is lodged in the left ureter.

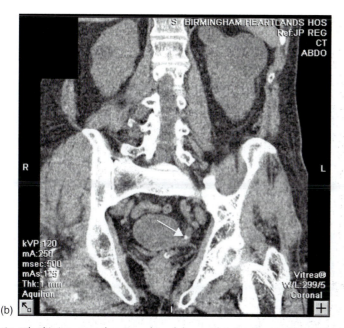

(b)

Fig. E5b. This is a coronal section of an abdomen showing the renal tract taken from a CT KUB study. This is done without intravenous contrast and enables visualization of the renal tract to identify renal stones. There is a small calculus seen at the lower end of the left ureter (see arrow). There is also a cyst seen in the left kidney in the mid pole.

Renal colic is a common problem. It is often due to a stone being stuck in the ureter with a dilated collecting system being present proximal to the site of obstruction.

Investigations

- Plain abdominal film kidney, ureter and bladder (KUB) – will reveal a small calcified stone often between 3 and 5 mm overlying the track of the ureter. Obstruction often occurs at the pelvic inlet or at the ureteric-vesical junction
- IVP – involves injection of intravenous contrast medium to demonstrate the kidneys and collecting systems. In a normal kidney and ureter contrast passes from the kidney down the ureter into the bladder in 5–10 min with no obstruction seen. Where there is a stone causing obstruction, back pressure builds up causing delayed renal excretion by the kidneys and often a dilated renal collecting system is seen to the level of the obstruction, best demonstrated on delayed films

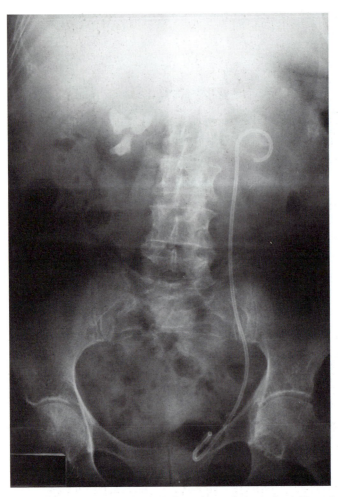

Fig. E6. Film demonstrating a large radio-opaque calculus in the right renal pelvis. The appearance is suspicious of a staghorn calculus on the right. A ureteric stent is noted in the left collecting system. The proximal end of the stent lies in the left renal pelvis and the distal end in the bladder.

CT KUB

This technique performed on the newer multi-slice CT scanners enables the renal tract to be visualized in both the axial and coronal plane without the need for intravenous contrast. Stones can be seen in the KUB and secondary signs such as perinephric stranding or hydronephrosis may be present.

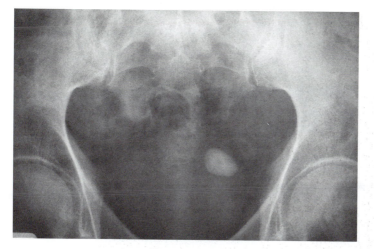

Fig. E7. Pelvic radiograph showing a large radio-opaque stone in the pelvis. The stone was in fact a bladder stone!

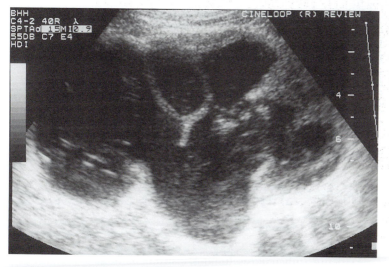

Fig. E8. Section taken from an ultrasound study of a patient's kidney. The black area within the kidney represents dilated calyces and a renal pelvis. This is the appearance of a hydronephrosis.

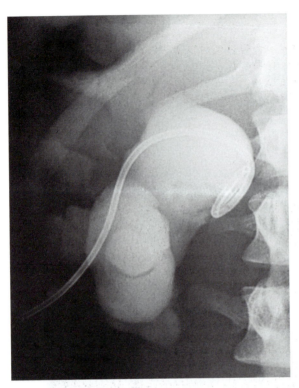

Fig. E9. Film showing the insertion of a nephrostomy into the dilated renal collecting system (which has been opacified with contrast).

Hydronephrosis

Renal tract obstruction (hydronephrosis) may be unilateral or bilateral.

Causes of unilateral hydronephrosis

- Pelvi-ureteric obstruction (PUJ)
- Stones in ureter
- Ureteric stricture (tuberculosis, tumour, instrumentation)
- Bladder tumour invading ureter
- Extrinsic mass, e.g. tumour from bowel, retroperitoneal fibrosis

Causes of bilateral hydronephrosis

- Prostatic outflow obstruction
- Pregnancy
- Retroperitoneal fibrosis/nodes

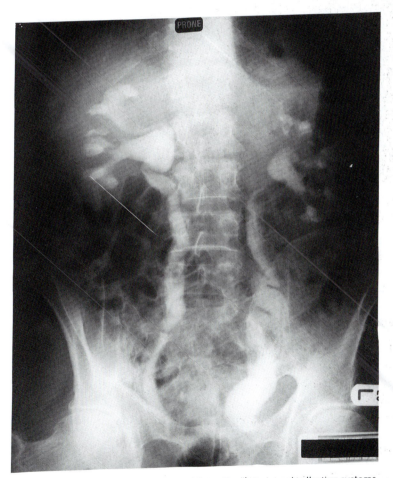

Investigations

- Ultrasound – demonstrates dilated renal pelvis and calyces may show distended ureter to level of obstruction
- IVP – delayed excretion of contrast in obstructed kidney eventual demonstration of dilated calyces, renal pelvis and ureter to level of obstruction

Fig. E10. Film from an IVP study showing bilaterally dilated renal collecting systems. Note the dilated left and right ureters. This patient had bilateral hydronephroses due to an enlarged prostate causing bladder outlet obstruction.

The patient presented with a vague abdominal pain and had a right-sided abdominal mass on examination.

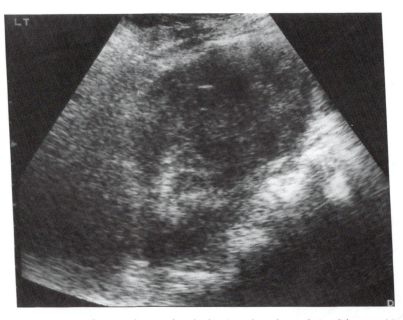

Fig. E11. Section from an ultrasound study showing a large hypoechoic solid mass arising from the upper pole of the kidney. The appearances are suspicious of a malignant tumour.

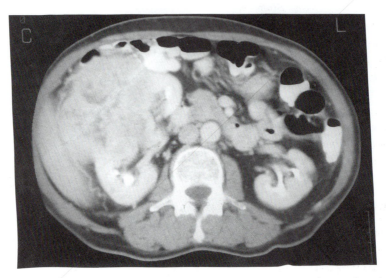

Fig. E12. Section from a CT study confirming the renal mass that is very large and causing extrinsic compression of the bowel. The IVC and renal vein do not appear to be involved by tumour.

Renal tumour

Ninety per cent of adult malignant renal tumours are renal cell carcinomas (10% are bilateral).

Other tumours

- Transitional cell (especially in renal pelvis, ureter)
- Squamous cell – associated with calculi
- Wilms (nephroblastoma) in children

Presenting signs

- Abdominal mass
- Pyrexia
- Haematuria
- Polycythaemia
- Metastatic symptoms

Radiology investigations

- Plain film of abdomen – amorphous calcification
- IVP
  - mass arising from kidney
  - distortion of calyces
  - non-functioning kidney
- Ultrasound – solid echogenic mass within kidney extending beyond surface when tumour is large
- CT
  - mass from kidney
  - extension into renal vein/intravenous catheter (IVC) can be assessed
  - nodes and metastases can also be seen for staging
- Chest radiograph – look for lung 'cannonball' metastases

Differential diagnosis of renal mass

- Abscess
- Haematoma
- Angiomyeolipoma
- Benign lesions, e.g. hamartoma

This patient presented with haematuria.

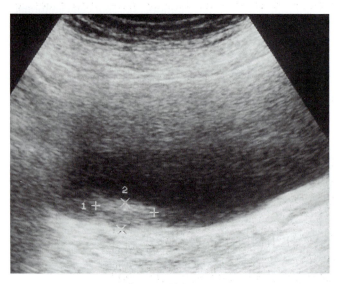

Fig. E13. Section from a bladder ultrasound study with the urine appearing black. Note the thickening in the bladder wall. This is highly suspicious of an early bladder carcinoma. A cystoscopy would be required to confirm this along with a biopsy of the area. In addition, a CT scan would be required to stage the bladder tumour for further treatment.

Bladder cancer

Bladder cancer is one of the commonest malignancies of the urogenital tract. It may present with haematuria. The histology is usually a transitional cell carcinoma. Bladder cancer is associated with:

- Smoking
- *Schistosoma haematobium* infection (squamous cell carcinoma)
- Chronic changes from bladder stones (squamous carcinoma)

Investigations

- Ultrasound – this may show bladder wall thickening
- IVP – may show filling defects in the bladder. If the tumour is involving the uretero-vesical junction there may be hydronephrosis present
- CT scan – can be used to stage bladder tumours. Invasion beyond the bladder wall and distant nodes can be assessed

- Chest radiograph – look for lung metastases
- Cystoscopy – mandatory in patients suspected to have bladder cancer. Direct inspection can be performed and tumours can be treated endoscopically by resection. In some cases cystectomy with ureteric diversion may be necessary

The patient presented with generalized abdominal swelling. A pelvic ultrasound was performed.

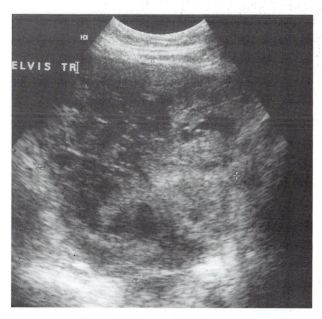

Fig. E14. Section from a pelvic ultrasound study demonstrating a thick-walled irregular cystic structure. The structure has solid and cystic components. In addition, there is some fluid around this area. This is an abnormal-looking ovary. The appearances are suggestive of carcinoma of the ovary. Further staging with a CT scan would be required.

Ovarian cancer

Ovarian cancer is a commonly encountered gynaecological malignancy. The tumour often presents late as early disease is often asymptomatic.

Investigations

- Ultrasound (trans-abdominal or transvaginal) – a pelvic mass is seen separate from the uterus. The tumour may be solid, cystic or both, the wall of the ovary may be thickened and septations may be present. Ascitic fluid may also be present (peritoneal metastases are common)
- CT/MRI – used for staging. The solid/cystic nature of the mass can be seen. Nodes can be identified; ascitic fluid, omental pathology can be seen

Common ovarian tumours

- Cystadenoma
- Cystadenocarcinoma
- Secondaries (Krukenberg tumours from stomach) (rare)
- Benign ovarian lesions
    - follicular cyst (thin-walled spontaneous regression)
    - corpus luteum cyst (in first trimester of pregnancy)

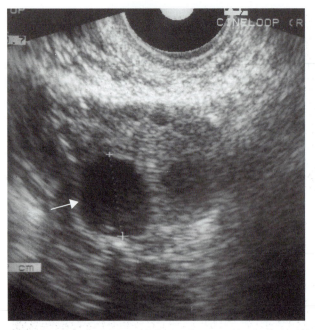

Fig. E15. Transvaginal scan of a normal ovary with a leading follicle present (see arrow).

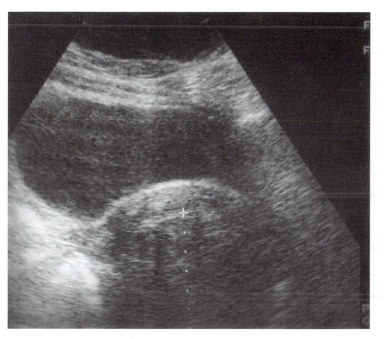

Fig. E16. Patient presented with heavy periods. The ultrasound examination shows an echogenic mass in the uterus that has the appearance of a fibroid.

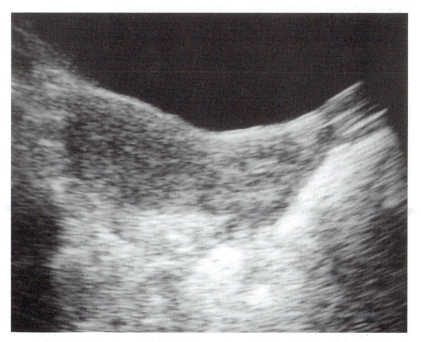

Fig. E17. Scan of the normal uterus showing a normal midline endometrial echo.

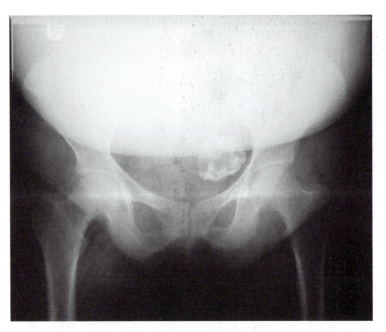

Fig. E18. Pelvic radiograph showing a calcified fibroid in another patient. Note the apron of fat in this patient who is obese.

Fibroids

The commonest gynaecological tumour is a fibroid. This is a benign tumour (leiomyoma) of the uterine smooth muscle. The uterus can be imaged using either trans-abdominal or transvaginal ultrasound. Trans-abdominal scanning requires a full bladder. Transvaginal scanning requires an empty bladder and the probe is introduced into the vagina.

Ultrasound features

- Hypoechoic mass arising from myometrium
- Echogenic areas may be seen if calcific degeneration is present

Other tumours that can be diagnosed with pelvic ultrasound

- Ovarian carcinoma – echogenic mass in pelvic adnexa separate from uterus
- Endometrial carcinoma – increase in the diameter of the endometrial echo (>7 mm) especially in the post-menopausal woman

Cancer of the cervix is best diagnosed early on smears. Staging of this tumour is best carried out using MRI.

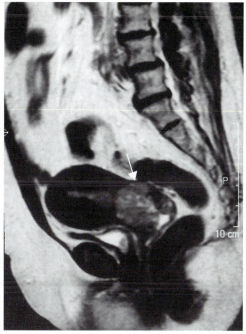

(a)

Fig. E19a. Sagittal T2-weighted MRI scan of the pelvis showing an abnormal signal mass in the cervix suspicious of a large cervical tumour (see arrow).

Obstetric scans

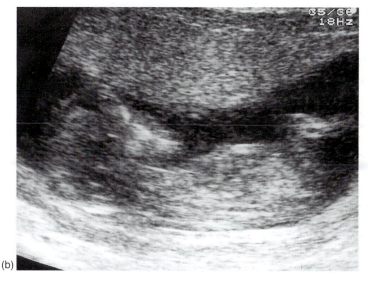

(b)

Fig. E19b. Scan showing an early intra-uterine gestation with the head, body and legs of the developing foetus identifiable. The scan has been performed trans-abdominally.

Ultrasound has revolutionized the way in which pregnancy is monitored. The purpose of antenatal scanning is to assess foetal position and viability, and also to identify malformations. In very early pregnancy, a detailed visualization of the gestation sac and foetal pole is possible using transvaginal scanning (the probe is inserted into the vagina).

Common foetal anomalies diagnosed antenatally

- CNS
  - hydrocephalus
  - neural tube defects
  - cleft palate
- Thorax
  - congenital diaphragmatic hernia
  - cardiac defects, e.g. VSD, ASD, Fallot's, etc.
- Abdomen
  - omphalocoele
  - intestinal atresia
  - renal defects, e.g. renal agenesis, polycystic kidneys
- Limb defects – hydrops foetalis

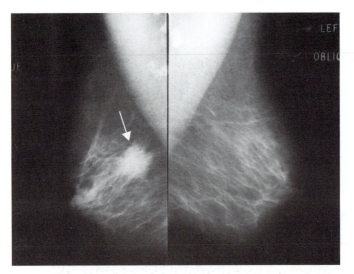

Fig. E20. Patient presenting with a right-sided breast lump. This is a mammogram. Note the area of increased density that has a spiculated border. This has the appearance of a carcinoma in the right breast. A few nodes are noted in the axillary tails on these oblique projections (see arrow).

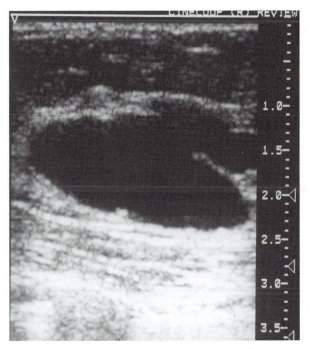

Fig. E21. Ultrasound of a breast showing a fluid-filled, well-defined smooth structure. This has the appearance of a cyst. The cyst can be aspirated and fluid can be examined to confirm the absence of malignant cells.

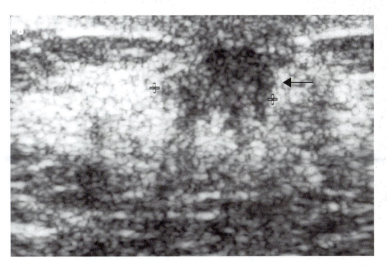

Fig. E22. Ultrasound of a breast showing an irregular hypoechoic mass underneath the skin suspicious of a cancer. Crosses show extent of tumour (see arrow).

Mammography

Mammography is the X-ray examination of the breasts. The breasts are compressed and craniocaudal and lateral oblique views are taken. The density of the breasts varies throughout a woman's life, the breasts being predominantly glandular in the young and fatty as one gets older. Glandular breasts are dense on mammography and, therefore, cancers are difficult to see in this group. Ultrasound examination is usually performed in younger women.

Signs of carcinoma on mammography

- Spiculated dense mass
- Clustered microcalcification
- Architectural distortion of adjacent breast tissue
- Skin thickening

Signs of benign lesions

- Usually smooth and well defined
- Coarse (larger) calcification
- No spiculation or tissue distortion

Ultrasound can be used to distinguish between solid and cystic lesions. Remember that it is not always possible to distinguish benign masses from malignant lesions on mammography alone. Triple assessment is performed:

- Examination/palpation
- Imaging
- Fine-needle aspiration/biopsy

The patient presented with swelling in the leg following a long coach journey.
Section from an ultrasound study of the patient's veins. Note the echogenic thrombus seen within the femoral vein. This is the appearance of a thrombosis.

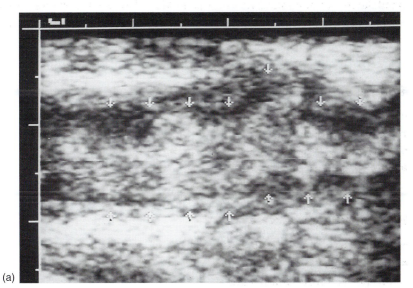

(a)

Fig. E23a. Longitudinal scan.

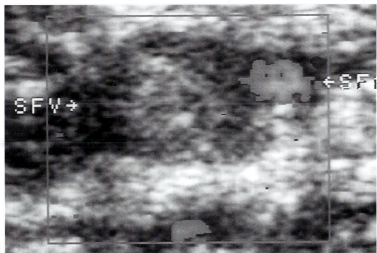

(b)

Fig. E23b. Transverse scan.

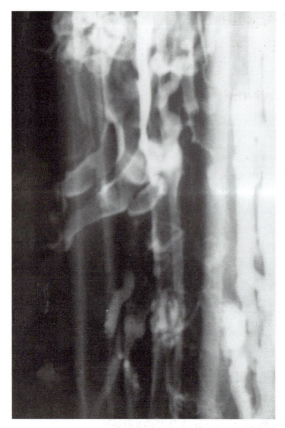

Fig. E24. Venogram showing filling defects in the calf veins caused by thrombi.

Deep vein thrombosis

Deep vein thrombosis is a common clinical problem. Clinical diagnosis is often inaccurate.

Presenting signs

- Calf pain
- Leg swelling
- Patient may present with signs of pulmonary embolus

Investigations (radiological)

- Compression Doppler ultrasound
- Venography

Signs on Doppler ultrasound

- Echogenic thrombus in the lumen of vein
- Vein not compressible
- Loss of venous flow pattern on Doppler

Doppler sonography is more accurate in femoral and popliteal vessels but less so in calf veins. Follow-up scans may help diagnose propagating thrombus.

Venography

Not usually performed as a first-line investigation. Involves injection of contrast medium into veins on the dorsum of the foot and following the flow of contrast up the leg.

The patient presented with abdominal pain radiating through to the back.

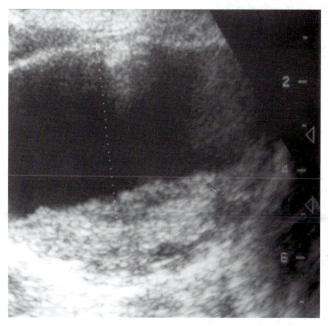

Fig. E25. Section from an ultrasound study showing a very dilated aorta. Note the echogenic thrombus on the posterior wall.

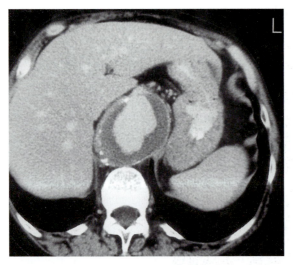

Fig. E26. CT section taken through the abdomen. This section of the study demonstrates the aorta, which is very dilated. The normal diameter should be <3 cm. A CT scan enables the visualization of calcification and thrombus within the aneurysm. In addition, it determines the length of the aneurysm and the site of origin and extent of the aneurysm. Using spiral CT scanning, the aorta can be reconstructed three-dimensionally enabling even better 3-D visualization of the aneurysm. This can help the surgeon plan for surgery.

Aortic aneurysm

An abdominal aortic aneurysm may present as an asymptomatic finding with a pulsatile mass with or without back pain. It may also present acutely with suspected rupture/leak and can mimic the symptoms of renal colic.

Investigation of suspected rupture

CT scan with intravenous contrast:
- Enlarged aorta
- Thrombus in walls
- Leak of contrast outside aorta
- Retroperitoneal haemorrhage
- Dissection flap

Investigation in asymptomatic patients

- Plain abdominal film – calcified walls of aorta may be seen
- Ultrasound – aortic diameter can be measured and the size can be followed up
- CT/MRI – can provide useful anatomical information about extent of aneurysm and involvement of renal/mesenteric vessels

Vascular intervention

A 70-year-old man presented with a history of sudden onset of pain in his right leg. What procedure has been performed and what does it show?

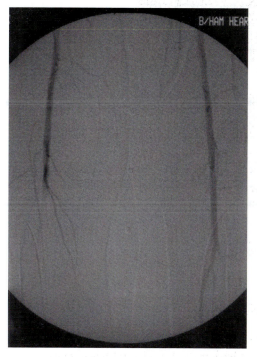

B/HAM HEAR

Fig. E27. Image taken from an arteriogram of the patient's lower limbs. A catheter has been introduced into the distal aorta via an arterial puncture of the femoral artery at the groin using the Seldinger technique. Contrast has been injected via a pump and images of the arterial vessels of the lower limb obtained to the level of the ankle. This frame shows a normal left popliteal artery with a good three-vessel run-off into the calf.

On the right there is an abrupt cut off noted in the popliteal artery with no filling of the tibial and peroneal vessels. Collateral vessels are noted at the knee. The features suggest an arterial embolus that is occluding blood flow beyond the right popliteal artery.

Management

- An embolectomy (surgical approach)
- Thrombolysis – catheter placed within thrombus and thrombolytic agents infused into it

- Catheter aspiration of thrombus
- Angioplasty if there is underlying stenosis of vessel
- Stenting can be considered in suitable cases

Other vascular procedures

- Angioplasty
- Insertion of tunnelled central venous lines for chemotherapy, etc.
- Stent insertion to keep narrowed vessels open
- Embolization of bleeding vessels and organs to stop haemorrhage
- Insertion of IVC filters to prevent pulmonary embolus in patients with significant femoral thrombosis
- Coiling arterio-venous malformations

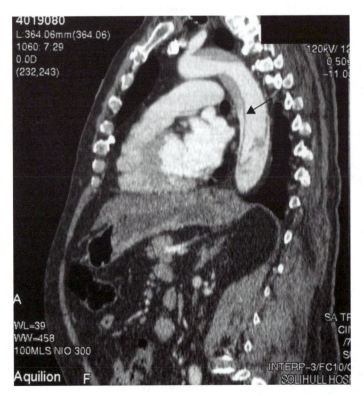

Fig. E28. This is a sagittal image taken from a multi-slice CT study of the aorta. This scan has been performed with intravenous contrast and shows the ascending and descending thoracic aorta. There is a dissection flap seen in the descending thoracic aorta with thrombus seen in the aortic arch. This is an example of a dissection of the aorta (see arrow).

Index